Study Guide to accompany

FOUNDATIONS AND CLINICAL APPLICATIONS OF NUTRITION: *A NURSING APPROACH*

Michele Grodner, EdD, CHES
William Paterson College

First Edition

This Student Study Guide is a companion to the first edition of *Foundations and Clinical Applications of Nutrition: A Nursing Approach*. The purpose of this guide is to provide a review of the major terms, concepts, and applications of nutrition from a nursing perspective. Each chapter highlights quotes of primary concepts from the text and is structured to provide a complete review and application of knowledge through specifically designs features. These features include:

Important Terms is a matching exercise of new terms and their definitions as applied to nursing and nutrition.

Applying Content Knowledge presents a practice clinical scenario based on the chapter topic to encourage critical thinking skills.

Quick Review features short answer questions, charts, matching, and fill-in exercises to provide a comprehensive review.

Practice Exam provides multiple choice questions to assist in testing preparation.

NCLEX Questions furnish sample questions based on the NCLEX nursing exam. Each chapter includes questions from the four NCLEX categories of physiologic needs (PN); safe, effective care environment (SE); health promotion/maintenance needs (HP); and psychosocial needs (PsN).

Answers to all review exercises and questions are included at the end of each chapter.

The reviewers, Joan Magee, of Henry Ford Community College, and Janet Azar, of Tidewater Community College, are to be commended for providing continuity of the evaluation process by reviewing both the text and this Student Study Guide. They were first and foremost concerned with ensuring that this Study Guide would be as useful as possible for students.

A final acknowledgment to Jean Babrick, Senior Developmental Editor, whose editorial suggestions and good humor greatly enhanced the educational value of this guide.

CONTENTS

Chapter 1 WELLNESS NUTRITION

"Wellness is a lifestyle through which we continually strive to enhance our level of health."

IMPORTANT TERMS

Write the terms from the list in the correct blanks on the right.

allowance

dietary standards

essential nutrients

health

lifestyle

nutrients

nutrition

precursor

Recommended Dietary Allowances

requirement

1. _____ nutrients that cannot be made by the body and must be provided by foods

2. _____ the amount of a nutrient needed to be consumed to maintain good health

3. _____ the merging and balance of five physical and psychological dimensions

4. _____ a guide to adequate nutrient intake levels against which to compare the nutrient values of foods consumed

5. _____ chemicals in foods that are required by the body for energy, growth, maintenance and/or repair

6. _____ the amount of a nutrient that must be consumed to prevent deficiency symptoms

7. _____ a pattern of behaviors

8. _____ average daily intake levels of essentials nutrients which meet the nutritional needs of almost all healthy individuals

9. _____ a substance that the human body can convert to a nutrient

10. _____ the study of essential nutrients and the processes by which nutrients are used by the body

1

APPLYING CONTENT KNOWLEDGE

" The goal of health promotion is to increase the level of health of individuals, families, groups, and communities."

       Health promotion strategies often involve lifestyle changes. Bob Ryan needs to reduce his dietary fat intake because he is at risk for coronary artery disease. He lives in a suburban community and takes a train into New York City where he works. Although it is only a half mile to the train station, he usually drives his car there to save time. Breakfast is often coffee with a midmorning coffee break providing Danish and more coffee; lunch is obtained from street vendors selling hot dogs and sausage sandwiches; dinner is usually eaten with his family but often features meat and potatoes, his favorites. Because he leaves early in the morning and returns tired in the evening, he says doesn't know how to change his behaviors.

       Using the strategies of knowledge, techniques, and community supports describe the education care plan that could be developed with him.

QUICK REVIEW

"An adequate eating pattern take into account assortment, balance, and nutrient density."

1.   What are three forms of education and where does each take place?

2.   Discuss the definitions of health used in the past and compare them to the present definition that is based on the dimensions of health.

3.   What is the role of nutrition in relation to the dimensions of health?

4.   From a nursing perspective, what is the goal of health promotion? Describe the function of knowledge, techniques, and community supports in achieving this goal.

5.   Describe the purpose and application of *Healthy People 2000*.

6.   Discuss the wellness approach towards nutrition.

7.   Define disease prevention and relate it to the classifications of primary, secondary and tertiary prevention.

8.   Compare undernutrition, overnutrition, and malnutrition.

9.   Explain the four components of nutritional assessment. Describe the potential

role of nurses in the assessment of nutritional status.

Categories of nutrients

"Nutrients are chemicals in food that are required by the body for energy, growth, maintenance and/or repair."

Match these nutrient categories, physiological roles, and energy values with their correct location on the following table:

indirectly assists other nutrients in energy release   4 kcal/gm
lipids   9 kcal/gm
major source of energy and fiber   0 kcal/gm
minerals   0 kcal/gm
serves structural purposes
source of essential fatty acids and fat soluble vitamins
water

Nutrient Category	Physiological Role	Energy value
carbohydrate	- (4) _____	4 kcal/gm
protein	- provides energy - many functions including structure of bones, muscles, enzymes, blood, immune system, and cell membranes	(8) __ kcal/gm
(1) _____	- most dense energy source - production of hormones - part of all cells - (5) _____	(9) __ kcal/gm
vitamins	_ (6) _____	(10) __ kcal/gm
(2)_____	- (7) _____ - affects the nature of fluids affecting muscles and central nervous system	0 kcal/gm

(3) _____	a major part of every tissue; constituent of blood; medium for chemical reactions and transportation of substances	(11) __ kcal/gm

Dietary Standards

"Dietary standards provide a guide of adequate nutrient intake levels against which to compare the nutrient values of foods consumed."

Using the terms provided, complete these statements:

access	deficiency	storage
allowances	prevent	supply
availability	recommendation	variations

1._____   4._____   7._____

2._____   5._____   8._____

3._____   6._____   9._____

Dietary standards are based on __(1.)__ for nutrients to provide for __(2.)__ in individuals needs and to supply enough for possible nutrient __(3.)__ in our bodies. Standards may be designed to provide the basic amount of a nutrient to prevent __(4.)__ symptoms or to supply sufficient amounts for basic good health. Levels of nutrients set may depend on the __(5.)__ of food in the country for which the standard is developed.

If easy __(6.)__ and plentiful __(7.)__ of foods are available, setting nutrient __(8.)__

higher than minimum is reasonable. If limited, the standard would be set to supply the

basic needs to __(9.)__ deficiencies.

Recommended Dietary Allowances

"The RDAs are average daily intake levels of essential nutrients that meet the nutritional needs of almost all healthy individuals."

1.   The RDAs recommend allowances for 19 nutrients. For each nutrient, 17 different levels are set based on age, gender and physiological needs of growth and pregnancy. In the table below fill in the boxes as to how these three characteristics affect nutrient intake levels.

Characteristic	Affect on nutrient intake needs
Age	(a.)
Gender	(b.)
Physiological needs (growth and pregnancy)	(c.)

2.   Below are 3 factors that are considered when RDA levels are set. In the space next to each factor give an example or explain how the factor influences recommended nutrient levels.

Factors	Example/Explanation
1. Average requirement and amount of variation	1.
2. Efficiency of use by the body	2.
3. Precursors	3.

3.   List 3 possible uses of the RDAs:

        1.

        2.

        3.

4.   Describe the purpose of the RDA margin of safety:

PRACTICE EXAM

1.   Education about health promotion takes place in the following form(s):
        A. formal
        B. nonformal
        C. informal
        D. a and c
        E. a, b, and c

2.   The primary role of nutrients is to:
        A. provide building blocks for the efficient functioning and
           maintenance of the body.
        B. provide energy and components of foods.
        C. maintain body fluid levels throughout the body.
        D. all of the above.
        E. none of the above.

3.   Health promotion increases the health level of:
        A. individuals.
        B. families.
        C. groups.
        D. communities.
        E. all of the above.

4.   Mary Steward has just been assigned to a community nursing position. She will
        be working with young children. Which one of the following documents should
        she consult to become familiar with nutrition priorities for American children?
        A. a nursing/medical dictionary
        B. Dietary Guidelines for Americans

C. *Healthy People 2000*
D. *Recommended Dietary Allowances*, 9th ed.
E. *Journal of American Dietetic Association*

5. Robert James is concerned about developing heart disease. He presently has no symptoms but asks you what he can do to prevent the development of coronary artery disease. The strategies you discuss with him are considered:
    A. primary prevention.
    B. secondary prevention.
    C. tertiary prevention.
    D. all of the above.
    E. none of the above because he has no symptoms.

6. As a home health care nurse, you are visiting Mrs. Maria Perez. She has just returned home from the hospital after being treated for diverticulitis. Both she and her daughter with whom she lives have questions about what Mrs. Perez can eat. You describe the purpose of her medical nutrition therapy developed by the hospital dietitian. The medical nutrition therapy or diet therapy is:
    A. primary prevention.
    B. secondary prevention.
    C. tertiary prevention.
    D. all of the above.
    E. none of the above.

7. Energy yielding nutrients include:
    A. carbohydrate, protein, and vitamins.
    B. minerals, water and lipid.
    C. protein, lipid, and vitamins.
    D. vitamins, carbohydrate, and minerals.
    E. lipid, protein, and carbohydrate.

8. Carbohydrate provides___ kcal/gm, protein ___ kcal/gm, and lipids___ kcal/gm, while alcohol provides___ kcal/gm.
    A. 4, 9, 7, 4
    B. 9, 7, 4, 4
    C. 4, 4, 9, 7
    D. 4, 4, 4, 7
    E. 4, 4, 7, 9

9. Protein is formed by the linking of:
    A. glucose in long chains of polysaccharides
    B. glycerol and fatty acids
    C. glucose and amino acids
    D. amino acids in various combinations

7

E. none of the above

10.   Essential amino acids are:
       A. only found in animal foods.
       B. found in animal and plant foods.
       C. only found in plant foods.
       D. only found in meat and chicken.
       E.   none of the above.

11.   The most dense form of energy is provided by:
       A. sucrose.
       B. fiber.
       C. lipids.
       D. alcohol.
       E. protein.

12.   All of the following are functions of lipids **except**:
       A. padding to protect body organs.
       B. provides dietary fiber.
       C. source of essential fatty acids.
       D. component of cell structure.
       E. production of hormones.

13.   The 3 categories of lipids are:
       A. saturated, monounsaturated, and polyunsaturated.
       B. lecithin, cholesterol, and sterols.
       C. glyceride, cholesterol and phospholipids.
       D. fatty acids, lecithin, and sterols.
       E. triglycerides, phospholipids, and sterols.

14.   Vitamins are divided into:
       A. names and numbers.
       B. 3 classes of saturated, monounsaturated, and polyunsaturated vitamins.
       C. 2 classes of monoglyceride and triglyceride vitamins.
       D. 2 classes of water soluble and fat soluble vitamins.
       E. 3 classes of major and trace vitamins.

15.   Each vitamin:
       A. serves several different regulatory functions.
       B. has a very specific metabolic function.
       C. is very flexible and can replace other vitamins.
       D. can be transformed into another vitamin.
       E. has a natural precursor in foods.

16. Functions of minerals include:
    A. a structural purpose as in bones and teeth.
    B. affecting the nature of body fluids.
    C. providing 4 kcal/gm.
    D. A and B
    E. A and C

17. Because water is a major part of every tissue of the body, we:
    A. can go weeks without water.
    B. can only live a few days without water.
    C. drink a few cups a day.
    D. should drink 8 - 10 cups a day of clear beverages.
    E. B and D

18. The RDA are:
    A. average daily recommended levels of essential nutrients for most
       healthy people.
    B. amounts of nutrients required to restore health after major illness.
    C. able to meet the nutrient needs of 10% of the population.
    D. only for individuals between the ages of 24 and 50 years old.
    E. essential nutrients for times of growth only.

19. Assessment of dietary intake may include:
    A. 24- hour recall.
    B. diet history.
    C. a food record.
    D. computer dietary analysis.
    E. all of the above.

20. Methods of assessing nutrition status may include:
    A. dietary evaluation.
    B. clinical examination.
    C. biochemical analysis.
    D. anthropometric measurement.
    E. all of the above.

NCLEX Questions

1. _____ provides the most efficient form of energy for the body especially   (PN)
   for muscles and the brain.
    A. sucrose
    B. glucose
    C. lipids

D. protein
E. amino acids

2. An example of a technique for health promotion is: (SE)
    A. teaching a young mother safe food preparation skills.
    B. being aware that salmonella can be spread because of inadequate food preparation skills.
    C. labeling of fresh poultry packages with information about proper food storage.
    D. watching a television show expose about industry errors in food processing.
    E. all of the above.

3. An example of knowledge for health promotion is: (HP)
    A. teaching a teenager how to choose healthier foods at fast food restaurants.
    B. information about the relationship of dietary intake and diet-related disorders.
    C. local supermarkets expanding the availability of fresh fruits and vegetables.
    D. none of the above.
    E. all of the above.

4. The dimensions of health include: (PsN)
    A. financial, emotional, ethnic, spiritual, and mental.
    B. psychological, physical, anthropometric, and spiritual.
    C. physical and anthropometric.
    D. physical, intellectual, emotional, social, and spiritual.
    E. none of the above.

ANSWERS
Important Terms
1. essential
2. allowance
3. health
4. dietary standards
5. nutrients
6. requirement
7. lifestyle
8. RDA
9. precursor
10. nutrition

Applying Content Knowledge

An education care plan developed with Bob Ryan could include: for knowledge, suggestions of books or videos on the relationship between diet and disease and on the process for changing behaviors; for techniques , from the knowledge gained, he can choose 3 applications such as getting up earlier to walk to the train, bringing fruit for the morning coffee break and only having lunch 2 days a week from the street vendors; and for community supports, determining which restaurants near his work provide lower fat meals and locating street vendors that sell fresh fruit.

Quick Review

1. Three forms of education are formal in school settings; nonformal through organized teaching or learning events such as at hospitals or community centers; and informal educational experiences from casual activities such as television, newspapers, or magazines.

2. The definition of health in the past focused on the absence of illness. In contrast, the present definition of health is broader and understood as the merging and balance of the five dimensions of health (physical, emotional, social, intellectual, and spiritual); it focuses on wellness and health promotion.

3. Nutrition is related to the dimensions in the following ways: physical is based on nutrients to maintain health; intellectual capacity depends on nutrients to maintain brain and CNS; emotional health is reflected by eating habits and patterns; social is connected to food as a means of communication and spiritual may view sustenance as sacred.

4. The goal is to increase the health of individuals, families, groups, and/or communities through lifestyle changes. Knowledge, techniques, and community supports provide the information, skills, and means to adopt healthier behaviors.

5. The purpose is to outline national health promotion and disease prevention objectives for Americans. It provides priorities of nutrition objectives.

6. The wellness approach provides ways to organize lifestyles and behaviors to support food consumption to increase health status.

7. Disease prevention is the recognition of a danger to health that could be reduced or alleviated through specific actions or through changes in lifestyle behaviors. Primary prevention consists of actions to avert the initial development of a disease or poor health. Secondary prevention involves early detection to stop or reduce the effects of disease or illness. Tertiary prevention is to minimize additional complications of a disorder or to help in the return to health.

8. All three terms relate to imbalanced nutrient intake. Undernutrition is a state of eating too few nutrients and/or energy. Overnutrition is the consumption of too many nutrients and/or too much energy, while malnutrition is a general term for imbalanced nutrient and energy intake.

Categories of nutrients
1. lipids
2. minerals
3. water
6. indirectly assists other nutrients in energy release
7. serves structural purposes
8. 4

4. major source of energy and fiber   9. 9
5. source of essential fatty acids   10. 0
   and fat soluble vitamins   11. 0

Dietary Standards

1. allowances
2. variations
3. strategy
4. deficiency
5. availability
6. access
7. supply
8. recommendation
9. prevent

Recommended Dietary Allowances

1. a. increased nutrient intake needed for growth that lessens as we age
  b. after puberty, males develop more lean body mass than females, which affects nutrient needs
  c. increased nutrient needs for tissue formation of growth

2. 1. vitamin C average requirement is only 10 mg; to provide for variation, RDA set higher
  2. only 10% of the iron consumed in food is absorbed; inefficient use by the body.
  3. beta carotene is a precursor for vitamin A

3. 1. creating a dietary standard for government food assistance programs
  2. interpreting food consumption information of individuals and populations
  3. basis of meeting nutrition goals such as those of *Healthy People 2000*

4. The margin of safety provides an additional safety factor by setting the RDA 30% higher than most individual needs.

Practice Exam

1. E	5. A	9. D	13. E	17. E
2. A	6. C	10. B	14. D	18. A
3. E	7. E	11. C	15. B	19. E
4. C	8. C	12. B	16. D	20. E

NCLEX Questions

1. B   2. A   3. B   4. D

Chapter 2 PERSONAL AND COMMUNITY NUTRITION

"... a person's food behavior is influenced by personal factors as well as community issues affecting food availability, consumption and expenditure trends, consumer information and food safety."

IMPORTANT TERMS

Write the terms from the list in the correct blanks on the right.

Daily Reference Values

Daily Values

Delaney Clause

incidential additives

intentional food additives

locus of control

Reference Daily Intakes

1. _____ a set of daily nutrient and food constituents values for which there are no RDAs, includes fat, fiber, cholesterol, and sodium

2. _____ substances purposely added to food products during manufacturing

3. _____ a system for food labeling composed of two sets of reference values (Reference Daily Intakes and Daily Reference Values)

4. _____ a set of daily nutrient values for protein, vitamins and minerals based on allowances of the 1968 RDAs

5. _____ the 1958 Food Additives Amendment to the federal Food Drug and Cosmetic Act of 1938 that bans any intentional incidental additives food additive found to induce cancer in man or animal

6. _____ the perception of one's ability to control life events and experiences

7. _____ substances that inadvertently contaminate processed foods

APPLYING CONTENT KNOWLEDGE

"Food safety is influenced by community decisions and personal behaviors."

Jenny Mills is again visiting her primary health care provider for a "stomach virus." She has been seen several times for the same problem over the past few months. As the nurse conducting the intake interview, you wonder if she could have a recurring foodborne illness. What are three assessment questions you might ask her?

QUICK REVIEW

"As knowledge of the relationship between diet and disease increases, public health approaches to diet-related disease prevention are formulated to encourage selection of foods, not just for their nutrient and energy content, but with primary disease prevention value as well."

1. Discuss how food preferences, food choice, and food liking affects food selection.

2. Describe how nutrient excesses led to the development of dietary guidelines to improve public health nutrition.

3. List the Dietary Guidelines for Americans. Identify the diet-related diseases for which the guidelines are designed to prevent or reduce the risk of development.

4. Describe the Food Guide Pyramid and the 5-a-Day program.

5. Explain the Exchange Lists for Meal Planning.

6. Discuss criteria for evaluating future research.

7. Describe the implications of food consumption trends for the nutritional status of Americans.

8. Describe the purpose and basis of nutrition labeling of food products. Discuss how nutrition facts can be used to evaluate food products.

9. Discuss the differences of responsibilities for food safety of the larger community (government agencies) and of the individual consumer.

10. List three types of microorganisms, viruses, or parasites found in food and their characteristic effects when consumed.

11. Describe three strategies for reducing the risks of foodborne illness.

12. Describe three methods for preserving food (include irradiation).

Dietary Guidelines for Americans

"The nutritional status of our communities is a reflection of our individual health."

1. Recommendations from numerous studies point to the relationship of dietary intake to the development of several chronic diseases. The Dietary Guidelines for Americans was developed to address this issue. Match the following diseases with the guideline addressing that disease. (A disease may be used more than once.)

alcoholism	diabetes	obesity
cancer	heart disease (coronary artery disease)	osteoporosis
cirrhosis of the liver	hypertension	stroke

Dietary Guidelines for Americans	Chronic Diet-related Diseases
1. Eat a variety of foods	1.
2. Maintain healthy weight	2.
3. Choose a diet low in fat, saturated fat, and cholesterol	3.
4. Choose a diet with plenty of vegetables, fruits, and grain products	4.
5. Use sugars only in moderation	5.
6. Use salt and sodium only in moderation	6.
7. If you drink alcoholic beverages, do so in moderation	7.

Food Consumption Trends

"Knowledge of changing patterns of food consumption and awareness of the rationale for food purchasing decisions is useful as we assist patients to modify their individual dietary patterns."

Match these health implications with their correct location in the following table:

A. ↑ intake of fiber, complex carbohydrate, lower kcalorie
B. ↑ consumption of calcium; ↓ consumption of cholesterol and saturated fats
C. ↓ intake of cholesterol and saturated fats
D. ↓ intake of nutrient-dense beverages
E. ↓ consumption of more nutrient-dense foods
F. ↓ risk of diet-related disorders

       ↑ = increased consumption   ↓ = decreased consumption

Food category	Change in consumption	Health implications
Fruits and vegetables	↑	1._____
Cereals and grains	↑	2._____
Meat, poultry, and fish	↑ ↓ beef ↑ fresh/frozen fish	3._____
Dairy products	↑ ↓ whole milk ↑ frozen dairy products, cheese, and low-fat milk	4._____
Sweeteners	↑ ↓ cane/sugar beets ↑ corn sweeteners/ noncaloric sweeteners	5._____
Beverages	↑ soft drinks and juices ↓ alcohol, milk, and coffee	6._____

Food Guides: Food Guide Pyramid and 5-a-Day

"Since we think about what food to eat, rather than which nutrients, nutrient recommendations are most useful when translated to real food."

1. Food Guide Pyramid

"The Food Guide Pyramid is designed to help us follow most of the Dietary Guidelines for Americans."

Match these terms with their correct location in the Food Guide Pyramid:

2 - 3	candy	dry beans	lentils	poultry	veal
3 - 5	canned	fruits	milk	pudding	vegetable
11	cereal	ice cream	oils	rice	yogurt
breads	cheese	juices	olive	spaghetti	

Food Group	Servings	Foods
(1)___,(2)___, and (3)___	2 - 3	milk (whole, lowfat, skim) cheese, yogurt,(4)___, (5)___
Meat,(6)___ , fish, (9)___ , eggs, and nuts	(7)___	beef, pork, lamb, (8)___, chicken, fish, legumes ((10)___, chick peas, split peas), eggs
(11)___	2 - 4	fresh, (12)___, and/or cooked fruit, melons, fruit juices
Vegetables	(13)___	fresh (raw), canned and/or cooked vegetables, vegetable (14)___
(15)___ , cereals, (17)___ and pasta	6 -(16)___	bread, rolls, muffins, ready-to-eat and cooked (18)___, rice, (19)___ , macaroni
Fats, (20)___, and sweets	use sparingly	corn,(21)___, peanut and other (22)___ oils, margarine, butter,(23)___, chocolate

2. 5-a-Day

"By focusing only on fruits and vegetables, 5-a-Day becomes an easy way to decrease intake of fats since fruits and vegetables are naturally low in fat."

Create a day's eating plan implementing 5-a-Day:

PRACTICE EXAM

1.   Diet-related diseases include:
       A. coronary artery disease (heart disease)
       B. hypertension
       C. diabetes
       D. chicken pox
       E. A, B, and C

2.   Dietary Guidelines for Americans:
       A. contain RDA guidelines.
       B. address national goals to reduce chronic diet-related diseases.
       C. address only coronary artery disease.
       D. focus on vitamin deficiencies of Americans.
       E. provides specific number of servings of food groups.

3.   The Food Guide Pyramid is designed to:
       A. assist in the application of the Dietary Guidelines for Americans.
       B. outline amounts and kinds of food to eat to maintain health.
       C. reduce risk of developing diet-related diseases.
       D. A and B
       E. A, B, and C

4. The Exchange Lists for Meal Planning list serving sizes that are similar
   in amounts of:
   A. fats and kcalories.
   B. carbohydrates and fiber.
   C. carbohydrates, fiber, and protein.
   D. fat and kcalories.
   E. carbohydrates, protein, fat, and kcalories.

5. Reference Daily Intakes (RDI) set standards based on the U.S. RDA for:
   A. protein, vitamins, and minerals.
   B. fiber, cholesterol, and lipids.
   C. fat, fiber, cholesterol, and sodium.
   D. fat, protein, and minerals.
   E. fiber, sodium, and kcalories.

6. Daily Reference Values are based on:
   A. protein, vitamins, and minerals.
   B. fiber, cholesterol, and lipids.
   C. fat, fiber, cholesterol, and sodium.
   D. fat, protein, and minerals.
   E. fiber, sodium, and kcalories.

7. Daily Values are based on two sets of reference values:
   A. Recommended Dietary Intakes and Daily Reference Values
   B. Reference Daily Intakes and Daily Reference Values
   C. U.S. RDA and Reference Daily Intakes
   D. Daily Reference Values and RDAs
   E. none of the above

8. Health claims on food labels that relate a nutrient or food to risk of a disease or
   health-related condition must:
   A. be decided upon by the manufacturers.
   B. apply to coronary artery disease and cancer.
   C. only relate to coronary artery disease.
   D. have FDA approval.
   E. be generally known to be true.

9. In order to have a safe food supply, it is essential that _____ be followed by
   each sector of the food chain.
   A. correct food handling procedures
   B. nutrient quantities of foods
   C. regulations by manufacturers
   D. food cooking guidelines
   E. none of the above

10. The primary approaches to setting risk standards for food safety are based on keeping certain substances out of the food supply. These approaches include:
    A. the "no significant risk" standard of California.
    B. the "zero risk" standard of the Delaney Clause.
    C. the "de minimus" standard.
    D. the "risk-benefit" standard of FIFRA.
    E. all of the above.

11. When the Delaney Clause went into effect, additives that were already being used and were considered safe were put on a:
    A. Generally in Use (GU) List.
    B. Recognized as Not Dangerous (RND) List.
    C. Generally Recognized As Safe (GRAS) List.
    D. Recommended for Safety in Consumption (RSC) List.
    E. Generally Regarded Additives (GRA) List.

12. Food additive regulation is supervised by the:
    A. National Academy of Health.
    B. American Medical Association.
    C. American Dietetic Association
    D. Food and Drug Administration.

13. *Salmonella* bacteria can be spread from:
    A. raw eggs.
    B. poultry.
    C. meats.
    D. cross-contamination.
    E. all of the above.

14. Symptoms of *Escherichia coli* may differ with each strain but most frequent symptoms include:
    A. bloody diarrhea.
    B. kidney problems.
    C. cramps.
    D. fevers.
    E. all of the above.

NCLEX Questions
1. Cooking acidic foods in cast iron skillets increases the iron content   (PN) of the foods prepared. This is an example of :
    A. an incidental food additive.
    B. an intentional food additive.
    C. a food safety hazard.
    D. a foodborne illness.

2. To prevent exposure to *Escherichia coli*, all of the following precautions   (SE) should be implemented **except**:
   A. cook ground beef to the well-done stage.
   B. do not eat any undercooked meat or poultry with any red or pink color.
   C. avoid cross-contamination between raw meats and other foods on cutting boards and surfaces.
   D. consume rare hamburgers only at home.
   E. observe all sanitary food handling procedures.

3. By adopting 5-a-Day, all the following will occur **except**:   (HB)
   A. decreased intake of fats.
   B. increased intake of fiber, vitamin C, and beta carotene.
   C. intake of the minimum number of fruit and vegetable categories of the Food Guide Pyramid.
   D. higher intake of grains, rice and pasta.
   E. the goals of Dietary Guidelines for Americans and *Healthy People 2000* can be achieved.

4. Sarah Smith, a young mother, is concerned about her young children's   (PsN) constant requests for high fat, sugary foods. She asks you for advice about how to change their food preferences. Which factor(s) might you discuss with her?
   A. genetic factor of preference for salty tastes
   B. environmental effect of parental food choices
   C. environmental effects of television watching
   D. their weight when they were born and their weight now
   E. B and C

21

ANSWERS

Important Terms

1. Daily Reference Values
2. intentional food additive
3. Daily Values
4. Reference Daily Intakes
5. Delaney Clause
6. locus of control
7. incidental food additives

Applying Content Knowledge

Assessment questions might include: Where do you eat most of your meals? How are the meals prepared? (follow up with related questions of food safety in food preparation such as are separate utensils and cutting boards used for raw chicken and beef?) Are foods left our unrefrigerated? For example, if she brings lunch to work, is a cold pack used or is a refrigerator available? Are foods such as soups and thawing meat left out overnight or allowed to cool for several or more hours before being cooked or refrigerated?

Quick Review

1. Food preference, food choice and food liking all affect our individual food selections. Food preferences are influenced by genetic determinants and environmental effects. Food choices are decided by factors occurring as we are ready to make specific decisions regarding which foods are available. Cost and convenience are prime influences. Food liking takes into account the foods we really like to eat without regard to any other factor besides taste. As we eat we weigh all these factors; we do have the power to weigh each differently to affect our nutritional status.

2. As nutrient deficiencies decreased, it was noticed that certain chronic diseases were increasing. Research revealed that there might be a relationship between dietary intake and the development of these diseases. Consequently, recommendations or guidelines to modify food intake were created to address this health issue.

3. The Dietary Guidelines for Americans are: 1. Eat a variety of foods; 2. Maintain healthy weight; 3. Choose a diet low in fat, saturated fat, and cholesterol; 4. Choose a diet with plenty of vegetables, fruits, and grain products; 5. Use sugars only in moderation; 6. Use salt and sodium only in moderation; 7. If you drink alcoholic beverages, do so in moderation .

Diet-related diseases may include heart disease (coronary artery disease), diabetes, cancer, hypertension, liver cirrhosis and obesity.

4. The Food Guide Pyramid, created by the USDA, divides foods into 5 major food groups of bread, cereal, rice and pasta; vegetables; fruits; milk, yogurt and cheese; meat and meat substitutes; and fats, oils and sweets as a group to be eaten sparingly. For each, the number of servings are given in a range. These types of food are needed to maintain health and reduce the risk of diet-related disorders. By following the Pyramid, most of the Dietary Guidelines for Americans are implemented.

The 5 a Day program created by the National Cancer Institute/National Institutes of Health and the Produce for Better Health Foundation is designed to increase our intake of fruits and vegetables to at least 5 a day. This allows for the implementation of several of the dietary recommendations.

5. The Exchange List for Meal Planning is a resource for serving sizes by dividing food into three different lists: carbohydrates, meat and meat substitutes, and fats. Each contains serving sizes of foods within that group a and each provides similar amount of carbohydrates, protein, fat and kcalories. It was first created by the American Diabetes Association and the American Dietetic Association for use by individuals with diabetes.

6. Criteria for evaluating future research provide an approach for assessing which recommendations should be implemented. They include 1) considering the source of nutrition advice, 2) assessing the comprehensiveness of the recommendations, 3) evaluating the basis of the recommendations, and 4)

estimating the ease of application.

7. Implications of food consumption trends are that they can affect nutrition status depending on the increase or decrease of certain food categories. If nurses have an awareness of these trends, they will understand the ease or difficulty of implementing new dietary recommendations.

8. The purpose of nutrition labeling is to provide consumers with nutrition information about products. Labeling is presently based on Daily Values which includes Daily Reference Values and Reference Daily Intakes. Nutrition facts can be used to identify the content of individual products or to compare products. If specific health problems are related to nutrient intake, such as sodium and hypertension, the amounts in food are easy to quantify.

9. It is the responsibility of the larger community to supervise the production and preparation of food products so that safety is assured at point of purchase. The responsibility of the individual consumer takes over once food is purchased when we have the obligation to properly handle food to prevent foodborne illness in the home through proper storage and preparation techniques.

10. 1) *Salmonella* appears 12-24 hours after eating with nausea and vomiting, cramps, diarrhea, chills, and fever. *2) Vibrio parahaemolyticus* appears 2-48 hours with flu-like symptoms and *3) Listeria monocytogenes* appears 1-12 days with flu-like symptoms that may lead to meningitis or an infection similar to mononucleosis.

11. 1) Do not place cooked foods on unwashed surfaces on which raw food has been prepared. 2) Never use a recipe that has raw eggs in it that are not cooked before eating. 3) Never buy or use foods in bulging cans, cracked jars, or with bulging lids. Botulism in the contents of contaminated food may cause the bulging of cans or lids or the toxin may enter through damaged openings. It is extremely toxic.

12. Three methods of preservation are canning, by which heat destroys microorganisms; refrigeration and freezing which restrict the growth of microorganisms by cold temperature; and irradiation, by which exposure to gamma irradiation destroys microorganisms, insects, and parasites that can spoil food or cause illness.

Dietary Guidelines for Americans

1. all diseases
2. all diseases
3. cancer, heart disease, obesity, stroke
4. all diseases
5. obesity, heart disease, and diabetes (weight-related)
6. hypertension, heart disease, stroke
7. alcoholism, cirrhosis of the liver

Food Guides: Food Guide Pyramid and 5-a-Day

1. Food Guide Pyramid:

1. milk	5. pudding	9. dry beans	13. 3-5	17. rice	21. olive
2. yogurt	6. poultry	10. lentils	14. juices	18. cereal	22. vegetable
3. cheese	7. 2-3	11. fruits	15. bread	19. spaghetti	23. candy
4. ice cream	8. veal	12. canned	16. 11	20. oils	

2. 5-a-Day:

Breakfast: oatmeal with banana (1)

Lunch: hero sandwich with lettuce and tomatoes(2)

Dinner: salmon florentine (with spinach) (3), baked potato (4), and salad (5)

Snacks: pear with cheese(6)
fruit with yogurt(7)

Food Consumption Trends

1. F   2. A   3. C   4. B   5. E   6. D

Practice Exam

1. E   3. E   5. A   7. B   9. A   11. C   13. E
2. B   4. E   6. C   8. D   10. E   12. D   14. E

NCLEX Questions

1. A   2. D   3. D   4. E

Chapter 3 DIGESTION, ABSORPTION, AND METABOLISM

"The health of the body is based on the nutrients available to support growth, maintenance and energy needs. The digestive system, responsible for processing foods, is itself dependent on our nutrient intake for its maintenance."

IMPORTANT TERMS

Write the terms from the list in the correct blanks on the right.

bile

bolus

chyme

constipation

diarrhea

digestion

gastrointestinal (GI) tract

lactose intolerance

peristalsis

segmentation

vomiting

1._____ the main organs of the digestive system forming a tube that runs from mouth to anus

2._____ the process through which foods are broken down into smaller and smaller units to prepare nutrients for absorption

3.._____ the rhythmic contractions of muscles causing wave-like motions moving food down the GI tract

4. _____ the forward and backward muscular muscular action that assists in controlling food mass movement through the GI tract

5._____ a masticated lump or ball of food ready to be swallowed

6._____ a semi- liquid mixture of food mass

7._____ a substance that emulsifies to aid the digestion of lipids; produced by the liver and stored in the gallbladder

8._____ reverse peristalsis

9._____ the inability to break down lactose, the carbohydrate in milk

10._____straining to pass hard dry stools; slow movement of feces through the colon

11._____ frequent passing of loose, watery bowel movements

25

APPLYING CONTENT KNOWLEDGE

"Heartburn, fortunately, has nothing to do with the health of our hearts."

James Carroll, a senior at the local university, is completing his internship at the rock radio station, while continuing to work at his part-time job. Without any time to spare, he has been eating meals whenever he can, often from fast food restaurants. These meals are usually gobbled quickly in his car. Lately, though, he is feeling stressed out and is experiencing heartburn. List 3 lifestyle behaviors that he could change to possibly reduce heartburn.

QUICK REVIEW

"The coordination of four layers of muscles (mucosa, submucosa, muscularis, and serosa) provides the muscular action that controls the movement of food mass through the GI tract."

1.   Describe the function of the primary organs used in digestion.

2.   Explain the organs and mechanisms used for nutrient absorption.

3.   Describe the elimination process.

4.   Review the process of metabolism.

5.   Identify a common health problem related to the GI tract and lifestyle behaviors. List 3 prevention or treatment strategies.

Hormones and Digestion

"Regulating the release of gastric juices and enzymes are hormones."

Place the hormone in the appropriate space:

Hormone	cholecystokinin-pancreozymin (CCK)	gastrin	secretin
	_____	_____	_____
Origin	stomach mucosa	small intestine	small intestine
Action	increases release of gastric juices in response to stomach distention caused by food	causes pancreas to release bicarbonate to small intestine; bile release from gallbladder	initiates pancreatic exocrine secretions; activates bile release from gallbladder

26

Digestive Organ Functions

"Everything eaten is processed through the GI tract. The digestive system functions to prepare ingested nutrients for digestion and absorption as well as to protect against consumed microorganisms and toxic substances."

Match these terms with their correct location in the table below:

anus	completes digestion	produces bile to aid digestion
gallbladder	forms and stores feces	stores and concentrates bile
pancreas	HCL activates enzymes	stores and expels feces
salivary glands	limited absorption	stores vitamins and iron
	produces bicarbonates	transports food

Organ	Function
mouth	-- breaks up food particles
(1)_____	-- saliva moistens and lubricated food -- produces amylase that digests CHO
esophagus	-- (2)_____
stomach	-- stores and churns food -- (3)_____ , breaks up food, kills germs -- mucus protects stomach wall from acid -- (4)_____
(5)_____	-- hormones regulate blood glucose levels -- (6)_____ that neutralizes stomach acid
(7)_____	-- (8)_____
liver	-- breaks down and builds up many biological molecules -- (9)_____ -- destroys old blood cells -- destroys poisons -- (10)_____
small intestine	-- (11)_____ -- absorbs nutrients and most water
large intestine	-- reabsorbs some water, ions and vitamins -- (12)_____
rectum	-- (13)_____
(14)_____	-- opening for elimination of feces

Food Transit Times

"During the passage through the GI tract, more than 95% of carbohydrate, fat, and protein ingested is absorbed."

Match the length of time with the appropriate process or organ.

about 5 hours	depends on texture and quantity	9-16 hours
2-6 hours	16-27 hours	5-7 seconds

1. _____ Chewing and swallowing

2. _____ Esophagus

3. _____ Stomach

4. _____ Small intestine

5. _____ Large intestine

6. _____ Total time

PRACTICE EXAM

1. Digestion depends on:
   A. chemical action of enzymes and hormones.
   B. chemical action of hormones.
   C. mechanical digestion.
   D. combined muscular (mechanical) and chemical actions.

2. A flap of tissue that closes over the trachea to prevent the bolus from entering the lungs is the:
   A. esophagus.
   B. stomach.
   C. small intestine.
   D. epiglottis.

3. Sphincter muscles include all of the following **except** the:
   A. pylorus.
   B. cardiac.
   C. ileocecal valve.
   D. anus.
   E. gallbladder.

4.	The cardiac sphincter functions to:
	A. control the movement of bolus from the esophagus into the stomach.
	B. prevent acidic stomach contents from refluxing into the esophagus.
	C. separate the stomach and small intestine.
	D. A and B
	E. A and C

5.	The gastric mucosa of the stomach wall contains gastric pits with glands whose function is to:
	A. secrete bicarbonate to reduce acidity.
	B. secrete stomach acid, HCL.
	C. create gastric juice containing digestive enzymes.
	D. A and C
	E. B and C

6.	Mucus in the stomach:
	A. protects the stomach walls from the HCL.
	B. destroys toxins.
	C. stimulates peristalsis.
	D. assists bile function.
	E. A and B

7.	The actions of _____ slowly releases chyme into the _____ or upper portion of the small intestine.
	A. ileocecal valve, duodenum
	B. cardiac sphincter, ileum
	C. cardiac sphincter, cecum
	D. pyloric sphincter, duodenum
	E. pyloric sphincter, jejunum

8.	The walls of the small intestine are adapted for absorption by finger-like projections called_____. On these are hair-like projections called_____ .
	A. macro-vacuole, microvacuole
	B. villi, microvilli
	C. capillaries, microcapillaries
	D. intestinal branches, microbranches

9.	Final absorption of any available nutrients occurs in the:
	A. large intestine.
	B. small intestine.
	C. rectum.
	D. anus.
	E. gallbladder.

10. Bacteria in the large intestine produce _____ that are then absorbed.
    A. minerals
    B. protein
    C. several vitamins
    D. water

12. Transport processes for absorption include all of the following **except:**
    A. engulfing pinocytosis.
    B. energy dependent active transport.
    C. passive diffusion and osmosis.
    D. facilitated diffusion.
    E. peristalsis and segmentation.

13. Catabolism, a metabolic process, is the breakdown of food components into smaller molecular particles resulting in:
    A. the release of energy as heat.
    B. the formation of new cells.
    C. the release of chemical energy.
    D. A and B
    E. A and C

15. The metabolic process of anabolism includes:
    A. forming new cell structures.
    B. creating new substances like hormones and enzymes.
    C. releasing energy as heat and chemical energy.
    D. A and B
    E. A and C

16. Waste products are excreted by the:
    A. lungs, kidneys, or large intestine.
    B. lungs, kidneys, or gallbladder.
    C. lungs, large intestine or salivary glands.
    D. lungs, gallbladder, or salivary glands.

18. The following may cause flatus **except:**
    A. fermentation of indigestible carbohydrates as found in legumes.
    B. dehydration.
    C. swallowing excessive amounts of air from chewing foods too quickly.
    D. lactose intolerance.

NCLEX Questions

1.   The small intestine is the major site of: (PN)
      A. digestion.
      B. absorption.
      C. excretion.
      D. A and B
      E. A, B, and C

2.   Which of the following age group(s) is most at risk for dehydration from   (SE)
      diarrhea?
      A. infants
      B. children and teens
      C. adults
      D. elderly
      E. A and D

3.   To alleviate constipation, which of the following foods would be helpful?   (HP)
      A. whole wheat bread, hot dogs, ice cream, and wheat germ
      B. white bread, oatmeal, milk, and yogurt
      C. whole wheat bread, oatmeal bran cereal, apples, and broccoli
      D. chicken, fish, baked potatoes, and watermelon

4.   The following are ways to reduce heartburn **except**:   (PsN)
      A. avoid high fat meals.
      B. avoid "eating on the run".
      C. try to lay down after to meals to relax.
      D. wear clothing that does not restrict the waist and midriff.
      E. reduce consumption of chocolate, peppermints, spearmint, or alcohol.

ANSWERS

Important Terms

1. GI tract
2. digestion
3. peristalsis
4. segmentation
5. bolus
6. chyme
7. bile
8. vomiting
9. lactose intolerance
10. constipation
11. diarrhea

Applying Content Knowledge

Three lifestyle changes to possibly reduce heartburn include: 1) restructuring his schedule so there is more time to eat meals and to chew foods well; 2) reducing the fat content of foods eaten to aid digestion ; and 3) considering whether constipation or selection of certain foods and drinks such as chocolate, alcohol, peppermint or citrus fruits may be irritants.

Quick Review

1. The functions of the primary organs are as follows. The mouth is the site of both mechanical digestion, where food is broken into smaller pieces, and the beginning of the chemical digestion of starch. The strong muscle action of the stomach further breaks chyme down, mixing it with gastric juices. The small intestine completes digestion. Its structure of villi and microvilli is the site of most absorption of nutrients and water. In the large intestine final absorption of small amounts of water, ions, and some vitamins occurs, but the primary function of this organ is to form and store feces.

2. Nutrient absorption occurs primarily in the small intestine with a small amount of absorption in the large intestine. Four mechanisms function for absorption of nutrients. Passive diffusion and osmosis allows absorption when equal pressure on both sides of the intestinal wall lets molecules pass through the capillaries. Facilitated diffusion happens when nutrient molecules need support from specific proteins to pass through. Energy-dependent active transport is required when fluid pressures hamper uptake so a pumping mechanism that uses energy kicks in with the support of a special protein carrier. Engulfing pinocytosis occurs when a substance touches the villi membrane. The villi encircle the substance, allowing it to pass through to the circulatory system.

3. The elimination process is the means for removing accumulated waste from the body. This includes undigested substances such as fibers, fats that have combined with minerals, water, bacteria and mucus. When the accumulation distends the rectum, the reflex to defecate (expel feces from the body) occurs.

4. The process of metabolism includes catabolism and anabolism. Catabolism is the breakdown process of nutrients by which energy is released either as heat or as chemical energy. Anabolism is the build-up or synthesis process by which new substances are formed such as new cell structures or formation of new substances such as enzymes. Both processes take place at the same time inside cells.

5. A common GI tract problem is flatus. For flatus or intestinal gas, the following may be helpful 1) if fiber intake is being increased, increase slowly to avoid difficulty in digesting; 2) consider if lactose intolerance may be a cause by noting physical reactions after consuming milk; and 3) when eating, chew more slowly to avoid swallowing air along with food.

Hormones and Digestion

gastrin   secretin   CCK

Digestive Organ Functions

1. salivary glands
2. transports food
3. HCL activates enzymes
4. limited absorption
8. stores and concentrates bile
9. produces bile to aid digestion
10. stores vitamins and iron
11. complete digestion

5. pancreas
6. produces bicarbonates
7. gallbladder

12. forms and stores feces
13. stores and expels feces
14. anus

Food Transit Times
1. depends on texture and quantity
2. 5-7 seconds
3. 2-6 hours
4. about 5 hours
5. 9-16 hours
6. 16-27 hours

Practice Exam
1. D   3. E   5. E   7. D   9. A   11. E   13. A
2. D   4. D   6. A   8. B   10. E   12. D   14. B

NCLEX Questions
1. D   2. E   3. C   4. C

Chapter 4 CARBOHYDRATES

"All carbohydrates are organic compounds composed of carbon, hydrogen, and oxygen in the form of simple carbohydrates or sugars."

IMPORTANT TERMS

Write the terms from the list in the correct blanks on the right.

enrichment

epinephrine

glucagon

gluconeogenesis

glycogenesis

glycogenolysis

insulin

phenylketonuria (PKU)

somatostatin

steroid hormones

thyroxine

1._____ a genetic disorder in which the body cannot breakdown excess phenylalanine

2._____ returning nutrients that were lost because of processing to their original levels

3._____ conversion of glucose to glycogen

4._____ conversion of glycogen to glucose

5._____ the process producing glucose from fat and protein

6._____ a hormone produced by the pancreas that regulates blood glucose levels

7._____ a pancreatic hormone that releases glycogen from the liver

8._____ a hormone produced by the pancreas pancreas and hypothalamus that inhibits insulin and glucagon

9._____ an adrenal gland hormone that enhances the fast conversion of liver glycogen to glucose

10._____ an adrenal gland hormone that functions against insulin promoting glucose formation from protein

11._____ a thyroid hormone affecting blood glucose levels by increasing glucose absorption and releasing epinephrine

APPLYING CONTENT KNOWLEDGE

"Although fiber 'passes through' our bodies without providing kcalories or nutrients, its texture provides bulk which thickens chyme and eases the work of the gastrointestinal (GI) muscles to regulate the movement of the food mass."

You are at a restaurant having lunch with friends. After hearing you order a sandwich on whole wheat bread, a friend comments, "Whole wheat bread, white bread, what's the big deal? They're all complex carbohydrates!" How would you respond?

QUICK REVIEW

"Increased levels of complex carbohydrates appear to reduce risk factor of chronic diet-related disorders such as heart disease, diabetes, and some cancers."

1.   Describe the classifications and structures of monosaccharides, disaccharides, and polysaccarides, and dietary fiber. List two food sources for each.

2.   Discuss these 3 issues of concern about sugar: sources in the food supply, consumption levels and health effects.

3.   Discuss the role of sugar alcohols and alternate sweeteners.

4.   Explain 3 health benefits of dietary fiber.

5.   Identify the functions of carbohydrates as an energy source in the body.

6.   Explain carbohydrate metabolism through blood glucose regulation.

7.   Define hypoglycemia. List 3 possible causes for hypoglycemia.

8.   Define diabetes mellitus. Briefly describe the 3 categories of diabetes mellitus.

Fiber

"Dietary fiber actually refers to several kinds of carbohydrate substances from different plant sources; all serve similar functions in the body."

Match these terms with their correct location in the table below:

apples	hemicellulose	pectin
citrus fruits	larger softer stools	popcorn
guar	lipids and cholesterol	whole grains

	Soluble	**Insoluble**
Fibers	1._____, mucilage, 2._____,and other gums	cellulose,3._____, lignin
Food Examples	legumes, 4._____, pears, 5. _____, oatmeal	6._____, leafy green vegetables, brown rice, 7._____
Physical Effects (specific to fiber type)	binds 8._____ as moves through digestive tract; slows glucose absorption	9 _____

Health Benefits of Fiber

"All the health benefits of fiber improve the physical functioning of the human body."

Match the potential health benefit with the action of fiber on body functions.

colon cancer   diverticular disease

constipation   heart disease

diabetes control   weight control

POTENTIAL HEALTH BENEFIT   *ACTION OF FIBER*

Decreased risk of:

1._____   feel fuller; less food consumed; fiber replaces foods higher in fat/kcal.

2._____   bulkier stool

3._____   maintains muscular strength of GI tract reducing the risk of pocketing

4._____   increased intake of fiber decreases intake of fat (a risk factor); increased fiber decreases exposure to potential carcinogens

5._____   increased fiber decreases blood cholesterol and lipids levels by reducing dietary fat intake and by binding lipids and cholesterol for excretion

6._____   increased fiber (especially soluble fiber) slows glucose absorption

PRACTICE EXAM

1.   The process by which plants store energy from the sun is:
      A. biosynthesis.
      B. photosynthesis.
      C. thermogenesis.

D. adaptive thermogenesis.

2. Carbohydrates are composed of:
   A. carbon, hydrogen, and oxygen.
   B. carbon, hydrogen, nitrogen and oxygen.
   C. carbon, hydrogen, and phosphorus.
   D. carbon, hydrogen, and calcium.

3. Simple sugars or simple carbohydrates include:
   A. polysaccarides and monosaccharides.
   B. polysaccharides and disaccharides.
   C. monosaccharides and disaccharides.
   D. monosaccharides and monoglycerides.

4. Monosaccharides include:
   A. glucose, fructose, and galactose.
   B. glucose, sucrose, and galactose.
   C. glucose, sucrose, and fructose.
   D. glucose, fructose, and maltose.
   E. glucose, fructose, and lactose.

5. Disaccharides include:
   A. maltose, fructose, and lactose.
   B. maltose, glucose, and lactose.
   C. sucrose, glucose, and lactose.
   D. sucrose, maltose, and lactose.

6. Complex carbohydrates include:
   A. polysaccharides of starch, fiber, and glycogen.
   B. polysaccharides of glucose, fructose, and lactose.
   C. polysaccharides of starch, whole grains, and glycogen.
   D. monosaccharide of starch, fiber, and glycogen.

7. Glycogen is:
   A. is a good food source of complex carbohydrates.
   B. is only found in plant foods.
   C. is a source of energy in plant and animal foods.
   D. the storage form of carbohydrates in the liver and muscles.

8. Sugar alcohols are _____ sweeteners providing _____ kcalories per gram; they are naturally found in _____ and include sorbitol and mannitol.
   A. nutritive, 4, fruits
   B. artificial, 7, vegetables
   C. alternative, 9, fruits

39

D. nutritive, 4, fruits

9. An advantage to sugar alcohols is that:
   A. they contain less kcalories than carbohydrate sugars.
   B. they do not encourage the growth of bacteria in the mouth.
   C. they taste much sweeter than other sugars.
   D. they may cause fermentation in the intestinal tract.

10. Aspartame, an alternative sweetener, is formed:
    A. by the bonding of two triglycerides.
    B. by the bonding of two monosaccharides, glucose, and fructose.
    C. by the bonding of two amino acids, tryptophan, and histidine.
    D. by the bonding of two amino acids, aspartic acid, and phenylalanine.

11. Dietary fiber, a _____ and complex carbohydrate, cannot be digested by humans because _____.
    A. disaccharide, human digestive enzymes cannot break the bonds of plant fiber
    B. polysaccharide, human digestive enzymes cannot break the bonds of plant fiber
    C. polysaccharide, enzyme supplements are necessary
    D. starch, human digestive enzymes cannot break the bonds of plant fiber

12. Absorption of glucose depends on the:
    A. active transport pumping system.
    B. passive diffusion and osmosis.
    C. facilitated diffusion.
    D. engulfing pinocytosis.

13. When needed for energy, glycogen is broken down by enzymes to produce a surge of energy. This process is called:
    A. glucogenesis.
    B. glycogenesis.
    C. gluconeogenesis.
    D. glycogenolysis.

14. Two hormones, _____ and _____ produced by the pancreas, function to raise blood glucose levels.
    A. glucagon and somatostatin
    B. glycogen and somatostatin
    C. insulin and glucagon
    D. insulin and somatostatin

15. Insulin dependent diabetes mellitus (IDDM) can:
    A. be prevented by lifestyle changes.

B. not be prevented by dietary intake or lifestyle behaviors.

C. be related to family history and aging.

D. be associated with overweight and sedentary lifestyle.

16. If gestational diabetes mellitus is not controlled, the following may occur:

A. large fetus size

B. premature birth

C. pregnancy-induced hypertension

D. all of the above

NCLEX Questions

1. The recommended intake of dietary fiber is: (PN)

A. 30-45 grams a day.

B. 15-35 grams a day.

C. 5-20 grams a day.

D. 20-35 grams a day.

2. Joyce Jones has been experiencing constipation. Which food replacement (SE) would most help to reduce the constipation?

A. whole wheat bread instead of white bread

B. applesauce instead of a whole apple

C. orange instead of orange juice

D. popcorn instead of corn chips

3. Non-insulin dependent diabetes mellitus (NIDDM) may: (HP)

A. be prevented by lifestyle changes.

B. not be prevented by dietary intake or lifestyle behaviors.

C. be related to family history and age.

D. be associated with overweight and sedentary lifestyle.

E. A, C, and D

4. Tania Steele sometimes feels weak and anxious when she has to work (PsN) through her lunch hour and isn't able to eat. She should:

A. keep complex carbohydrate and protein snack foods available to reduce hyperglycemic symptoms.

B. keep complex carbohydrate and protein snack foods available to reduce hypoglycemic symptoms.

C. keep high fat and high fiber snack foods available to reduce hyperglycemic symptoms.

D. keep high fat and high fiber snack foods available to reduce hypoglycemic symptoms.

ANSWERS

Important Terms

1. phenylalanine (PKU)   3. glycogenesis   5. gluconeogenesis   7. glucagon   9. epinephrine
2. enrichment   4. glycogenolysis 6. insulin   8. somatostatin 10. steroid hormone
                                                                                  11. thyroxine

Applying Content Knowledge

Whole wheat bread and white bread are complex carbohydrates because they are composed of polysaccharides that are easily broken down to provide simple carbohydrates. The difference is that whole wheat bread also contains polysaccharides, fiber, that the human digestive system cannot break down; this fiber provides many potential health benefits as it passes through the GI tract. In addition, foods made from whole grains also contain more vitamins and minerals that are not restored to refined flours such as the white flour used to make white bread.

Quick Review

1. The two classifications of carbohydrates are called simple carbohydrates (monosaccharides and disaccharides) and complex carbohydrates (polysaccharides). All carbohydrates are composed of monosaccharides that are linked together. Monosaccharides are single carbohydrate units and include glucose, fructose, and galactose. Disaccharides are two single monosaccharides bound together. Sucrose, maltose, and lactose are disaccharides. Polysaccharides are formed from numerous monosaccharides bound together. Polysaccharides include starch, fiber, and glycogen. Dietary fiber cannot be broken down by human digestive juices and glycogen is a storage form of carbohydrate found only in the liver and muscles of live animals and humans. Two foods sources for each are: for monosaccharides, vegetables, and milk; for disaccharides, fruits and cheese; polysaccharides, grains and legumes.

2. Sources of sugar in the food supply are a concern because although they may come from a variety of sources they still only add kcalories and no other nutrients. Consumption levels are a concern because our overall intake of sweeteners has increased from the rise in use of high fructose corn syrup. This means that although our intake of refined white sugar has declined, our overall intake of sweets has increased. Finally, the potential health effects are that nutrient displacement can occur as sweet foods often replace foods of higher nutrient density such as skim milk being replaced by sweetened ice tea. Specifically sugar intake is only directly related to dental caries; sugar helps the growth of bacteria that can lead to plaque formation. Sugar intake may be tied to obesity if an excess of kcalories is consumed, but more often sweet foods tend to be high in fat and it is the kcalories from fat that provide the excess energy.

3. Sugar alcohols and alternate sweeteners provide another source of sweetness in addition to sucrose and fructose. Sugar alcohols include sorbitol, mannitol, and xylitol. Found naturally in fruits, they still provide 4 kcalories per gram, but reduce the risk of tooth decay. They are metabolized more slowly than other sugars because the GI tract needs more time to convert the sugar alcohol to glucose. Blood glucose levels are more slowly affected. A disadvantage is that large quantities of sugar alcohols may ferment during the digestive process causing diarrhea.

Alternative or artificial sweeteners are synthetically manufactured to provide sweetness with as few kcalories, if any, as possible. Aspartame, saccharin, and acesulfame potassium (K) are the most commonly used in the United States.

Aspartame is formed by bonding the amino acids aspartic acid and phenylalanine. When aspartame is digested, it is absorbed as the two amino acids. Because it is about 200 times as sweet as sucrose, very small quantities are needed so that the kcaloric value is minimal. Because it does not have an aftertaste, it has replaced saccharin in a variety of foods. Individuals with the genetic disorder of PKU should not consume products with aspartame because of the additional amount of phenylalanine provided.

Saccharin is up to 700 times as sweet as sucrose. Because saccharin has a bitter aftertaste, it is used in combination with other alternative sweeteners. It has been tied to possible bladder cancer, but Congressional legislation allows its use to continue.

Acesulfame K is about 200 times as sweet as sucrose and is not digested by the human body so it provides no kcalories. Its use is still limited. Individuals who need to restrict their potassium intake should seek advice regarding acceptable intake levels.

4. Three benefits of dietary fiber are that it reduces the risk of diverticular disease (maintains health of GI tract), colon cancer (removes potential carcinogenic substances quickly), and heart disease (binds triglycerides and cholesterol for excretion).

5. Carbohydrates provide the most efficient form of energy for the body. If fats are the predominate source of energy, ketones (by-products of fat metabolism) develop that stress body functions and may affect the pH levels of the body. Protein can also provide energy, but its use reduces the amount of protein available for specific protein functions. Consequently, the best source of energy is carbohydrates. This process allows protein to be spared and used for specific protein functions rather than for energy needs.

6. Maintaining blood glucose regulation is a primary function of carbohydrate metabolism. Homeostasis is achieved at a level between 70 to 120 mg/dL. Glucose is the sugar most available for energy in the blood. It may come from carbohydrate and non-carbohydrate sources. All carbohydrates that are consumed are eventually available as glucose (with the exception of dietary fiber which cannot be digested). Glycogen can be drawn from the liver and converted back to glucose through glycogenolysis. Other intermediate carbohydrate metabolites, such as lactic acid and pyruvic acid, are also available. Through gluconeogenesis, protein and fats can provide blood glucose but the process is not as efficient as using carbohydrates as the source of glucose.

7. Hypoglycemia occurs when blood glucose levels are below normal values. If a person hasn't eaten for a few hours, blood glucose levels get low and the body switches to alternate sources of energy such as stored liver glycogen. Sometimes this transition may be accompanied by anxiety, weakness, rapid heartbeat, and hunger. Hypoglycemia is not a disease, but represents symptoms of a disorder. Three possible causes for this may be an inadequate or erratic dietary intake pattern, over-production of insulin by the pancreas, or intestinal malabsorption of glucose.

8. Diabetes mellitus is a disorder of carbohydrate metabolism characterized by hyperglycemia caused by defective or deficient insulin. Three categories of diabetes are insulin-dependent diabetes mellitus (IDDM), non-insulin-dependent diabetes mellitus (NIDDM), and gestational diabetes mellitus (GDM). IDDM is a type of diabetes in which no insulin is produced by the pancreas; insulin is provided by daily injections. NIDDM is a form of diabetes in which some insulin is produced but it is defective and not able to serve the needs of the body; lifestyle changes and oral medications are used to control this disorder. Gestational diabetes occurs during pregnancy most commonly after the 20th week of gestation. The level of blood glucose remains abnormally high and may affect the health of the mother and of the fetus. Complications that may occur if blood glucose levels are not controlled include pregnancy-induced hypertension, premature birth, and large fetus size.

Fiber
1. pectin
2. guar
3. hemicellulose
4. apples
5. citrus fruits
6. whole grains
7. popcorn
8. lipids and cholesterol
9. larger stools

Health Benefits of Fiber
1. weight control
2. constipation
3. diverticular disease
4. colon cancer
5. heart disease
6. diabetes control

Practice Exam

1. B	4. A	7. D	10. D	13. D
2. A	5. D	8. A	11. B	14. A
3. C	6. A	9. B	12. A	15. B
				16. D

NCLEX Questions

1. D	2. A	3. E	4. A

Chapter 5 FATS

" Fats actually refer to the chemical group of lipids. Lipids are divided into three classification: fats or triglycerides and the fat -related substances of phospholipids and sterols."

IMPORTANT TERMS

Write the terms from the list in the correct blanks.

acetyl coenzyme A

adipose tissue

atherosclerosis

chylomicrons

eicosapentaenoic acid (EPA)

emulsifier

essential fatty acids

ketosis

lipogenesis

plaque

TCA cycle

1._____ a substance that works by being soluble in water and fat at the same time

2._____ polyunsaturated fatty acids that cannot be made in the body and must be consumed in the diet

3._____ stored form of fat (mainly triglycerides) in the body

4._____ the main omega-3 fatty acid in fish

5._____ deposits of fatty substances, including cholesterol, that attach to arterial walls

6._____ accumulation of plaques that results in blockage in the arteries

7._____ the first lipoproteins formed after absorption of lipids from food

8._____ important intermediate byproduct in metabolism formed from the breakdown of glucose, fatty acids, and certain amino acids

9._____ cellular reactions that liberate energy from fragments of carbohydrates, fats, and protein

10._____ a condition in which the absence of plasma glucose results in partial oxidation of fatty acids

11._____ anabolism (synthesis) of lipids

APPLYING CONTENT KNOWLEDGE

"Since we cannot control our heredity, the main goal for all, regardless of genes, is prevention to lower the risk factors for atherosclerosis and heart disease that are under our control."

Disease prevention for chronic diet-related diseases depends on changes in lifestyle behaviors. Consider the lifestyle behaviors John Mason could adopt based on his personal history. John Mason is a 20 year old Caucasian male; his mother and father both have high cholesterol levels and histories of coronary artery disease in their families. Although John's cholesterol level is average for his age, what three disease prevention strategies could he pursue? Would these strategies be primary, secondary or tertiary?

QUICK REVIEW

"The functions of lipids divide into two categories; some functions are through characteristics of lipids in foods and others are related to the physical health of our bodies."

1. List three functions of fats (triglycerides) in food and three physiological functions of fats (triglycerides).

2. Identify the essential fatty acids. Describe why they are essential and name two food sources.

3. Describe the structures and functions of phospholipids and sterols.

4. Explain preservation of fats and oils in foods. Discuss the roles hydrogenation and antioxidants.

5. Differentiate between food cholesterol and blood cholesterol. Explain the functions of VLDLs, LDLs, and HDLs and their relationships to the development of atherosclerosis.

6. Discuss the unique processes of fat absorption.

7. Lipid metabolism consists of several processes. Describe lipid catabolism and anabolism. List the hormones that regulate these processes.

8. Briefly review the possible relationship between dietary fat intake and the development of cancer, NIDDM, and hypertension.

Types of Fatty Acids

"All natural fats are mixtures of different types of fatty acid. Most plants oils contain some saturated fatty acids, and animal fats contain amounts of polyunsaturated fats. The predominate type of fat in a food determines its category."

Using the terms provided, complete this table.

↑ blood cholesterol   coconut   fish   shortening

↓ blood cholesterol   corn   olive   one unsaturated double bonds

canola oil   dairy products   palm   single bonded carbon chains

Category	saturated	monounsaturated	polyunsaturated
Structure	1 _____	2 _____	two or more unsaturated double bonds
Food sources	meats, 3. _____, animal fats, egg yolks, 4. _____, 5. _____ and 6. _____ oils	7. _____ oil, peanut butter, peanut oil, 8. _____ oil	oils of 9. _____, sunflower, sesame, safflower, and wheat germ, 10. _____, margarine
Health effects	11 _____	no effect on blood cholesterol	12 _____

Triglyceride Digestion

"...bile emulsifies fats to facilitate digestion."

Match these digestive actions and terms with their correct location below.

CCK   foods broken into smaller pieces   peristalsis
enzymes   glycerol   triglycerides
fatty acids hydrolyzed

Organ	Mechanical	Chemical
Mouth	1._____	none
Stomach	2._____	3._____ (lingual lipase, gastric lipase) triglycerides 4._____ to fatty acids
Small intestine	peristalsis	5._____ causes release of bile

chemical and mechanical allows pancreatic lipase to complete breakdown of 6._____ to 7._____, monoglycerides, 8._____

Large intestine	undigested fats exit in feces	

PRACTICE EXAM

1.   In addition to caloric content, fat also:
      A. contains essential fatty acids.
      B. transports fat soluble vitamins.
      C. contains water soluble vitamins.
      D. A and B

2.   Sterols are components of _____ and are need to make _____.
      A. triglycerides; energy and vitamin D
      B. triglycerides; bile, brain, and nerve tissue cells
      C. complex regulatory compounds; sex hormones, bile, vitamin D, and brain and nerve tissue cells
      D. complex regulatory compounds; gastric juices, vitamin A, and adipose cells

3.   A compound containing carbon, hydrogen, and oxygen with 3 fatty acids attached to a glycerol molecule is a:
      A. phospholipid.
      B. sterol.

C. monounsaturate.

D. triglyceride.

4. The level of saturation of a fat is determined by:
    A. the number of double bonds.
    B. the type of glycerol bonding.
    C. the number of side rings containing phosphates.
    D. the number of side rings containing nitrogen.

5. An essential lipid is:
    A. cholesterol.
    B. palmitic acid.
    C. lecithin.
    D. linoleic acid.

6. Based on a daily intake of 2,200 kcalories, how many kcalories and grams of fat should a female consume to meet the recommended 30% or less of kcalories per day?
    A. 330 kcal and 36 grams or less
    B. 330 kcal and 47 grams or less
    C. 660 kcal and 73 grams or less
    D. 660 kcal and 165 grams or less

7. Identifying the type of fatty acids contained in different dietary fats is important because:
    A. high intake of saturated fatty acids is associated with high blood cholesterol levels.
    B. different types of fatty acids contain varying amounts of kcalories.
    C. a low intake of saturated fats is associated with high blood cholesterol levels.
    D. a way to increase high-density lipoproteins is to exercise.

8. Ways to preserve fats in food include:
    A. hydrogenation to reduce saturation of fats and decrease risk of rancidity.
    B. oxidize fats by using natural (vitamins E and C) and synthetic antioxidants (BHT and BHA).
    C. use of natural (BHA and BHT) and synthetic antioxidants (vitamins E and C).
    D. hydrogenation to increase saturation of fats and reduce risk of rancidity.

9. After fat is absorbed, it enters the bloodstream by way of the:
    A. bile duct.
    B. portal vein.
    C. lymphatic system.
    D. A and B

10. Which lipoprotein should be increased to reduce risk of coronary artery disease?
    A. chylomicron
    B. very low-density lipoprotein
    C. low-density lipoprotein
    D. high-density lipoprotein

NCLEX Questions

1. Cases of failure to thrive can occur if the fat intake of infants   (PN)
   is overly-restricted. Infants and young children depend on _____ and _____
   for the formation of brain and nerve tissue.
   A. triglycerides; kcalories
   B. dietary fats; cholesterol
   C. dietary fats; carbohydrates
   D. dietary fats; vitamin D

2. Deficiencies of EPA may occur among: (SE)
   A. patients with fat malabsorption.
   B. elderly patients with peripheral vascular disease.
   C. patients recovering from serious burns.
   D. individuals with extremely low dietary fat intake.
   E. all of the above

3. Studies show that Americans most enjoy high fat foods. To introduce   (HP)
   health promoting snacking styles for children, which of the following snack
   platters accounts for the desire for fats while still meeting lower fat intake goals?
   A. fried corn puffs with apple slices
   B. carrot sticks with nonfat yogurt dip
   C. sliced apples and pears with thin cheese slices and lower fat crackers
      or lower fat taco chips
   D. no snacks served; three meals a day optimum

4. Freda Cooperman lived in a rural part of Russia where cooking with   (PSN)
   animal fats was common. Now in her eighties, she lives with her daughter's
   family in Boston, Massachusetts. She has just learned that she has coronary
   artery disease. Which would most meet her physical as well as psychological
   needs?
   A. advise her to only use margarine and vegetable oils instead of all animal fats
      and to only eat skinless breast of chicken and fish as animal foods
   B. discuss the ways she prepares the foods she most often eats and suggest ways
      to reduce the use of animal fats
   C. advise her to eat more fruits and vegetables and to consume less animals fats
      by replacing some of the fats with margarine and corn oil
   D. suggest that she adopt a low fat vegetarian dietary pattern..
   E. B and C

ANSWERS
Important Terms
1. emulsifier
2. essential fatty acids
3. adipose tissue
4. eicosapentaenoic (EFA)

5. plaque
6. atherosclersosis
7. chylomicrons
8. acetyl coenzyme A

9. TCA cycle
10. ketosis
11. lipogenesis

Applied Content Knowledge

Three strategies include 1) reduce intake of dietary cholesterol and saturated fats, 2) increase intake of fruits and vegetables, and 3) exercise regularly. These are primary prevention strategies.

Quick Review

1. Three functions of fats in foods are providing energy; carriers of vitamins A, D, E, and K and essential fatty acids; and creating palatability of taste. Three physiological functions are organ protection, body temperature regulator, and transmission of nerve impulses.

2. The essential fatty acids (EFA) are linoleic and linolenic fatty acids. These fatty acids are essential because they can't be manufactured by the body and must be consumed in the diet. EPA are required components of compounds such as prostaglandins and cell membranes. Vegetable oils are a primary source.

3. Phospholipids contain two fatty acids with a phosphate group attached to a backbone of glycerol. Functions include actions as a fat emulsifier and as a component of cell walls. Because they are manufactured by the body, phospholipids are not essential nutrients.

Sterols consist of carbon rings with side chains of carbon, hydrogen, and oxygen. Functions include part of complex regulatory compounds and a constituent of bile, vitamin D, sex and other hormones and cells in brain and nerve tissues. As with phospholipids, sterols are not essential nutrients because they are manufactured by the body.

4. Unsaturated fats in foods are more easily oxidized and then become rancid. Rancidity of fats changes their flavor, produces bad odors and possible illness. Hydrogenation, a process through which hydrogen is added to unsaturated fats, makes fats more stable and less at risk for rancidity. It also converts the unsaturated fatty acids of a fat to saturated lowering the health promotion values of fats that originally contained unsaturated fatty acids.

Antioxidants also reduce oxidation by blocking oxidation. Natural forms of oxidation include vitamin E (tocopherol) and C (ascorbic acid). Synthetic forms include butylated hydroxyanisole (BHA) and butylated hydroxytoluene (BHT).

5. Food cholesterol is the waxy lipid substance found in animal foods. When we consume food cholesterol, the body digests the dietary cholesterol. The liver uses the components of the cholesterol and saturated fatty acids to formulate new lipids. Blood cholesterol includes cholesterol formed by the liver that is distributed throughout the body. Blood cholesterol also includes cholesterol that has been discarded by cells and is traveling out of the body for either reuse or excretion. Very low-density lipoproteins are the first to leave the liver and contains quantities of cholesterol, triglycerides, and phospholipids. As the lipids circulate within the blood, fats are deposited for use by the cells of the body. As the density of the lipoprotein changes, they become low density lipoproteins (LDLs). LDLs may also deposit cholesterol along the artery walls as it continues through the bloodstream. These deposit can lead to the build-up of plagues and atherosclerosis. High density lipoproteins are considered "good cholesterol" because remove cholesterol from the cells for disposal by the liver.

6. In order for fats to be absorbed and travel through the circulatory system, micelles encircle the fat components to assist absorption. Once absorbed, fats reform to triglycerides. They are covered by protein

51

to be carried along with cholesterol and as chylomicrons enter the lymph system. From the lymph system, the absorbed fats enter the circulatory system and travel on to the liver.

7. Catabolism or breakdown of lipids provides two carbon units that are part of acetyl coenzyme A. Acetyl Co A enters the TCA cycle. If fat is used for energy, in the absence of carbohydrate, by-products of fat catabolism, ketone, accumulates. Lipogenesis or anabolism of lipids results in the formation of new triglycerides, phospholipids, cholesterol, and prostaglandins. Some of the triglycerides may be stored in adipose tissues. The component of these new lipids may be provided from foods other than fats.

Hormones that regulates these processes are insulin, growth hormone, adrenocorticotropic hormone, and glucocorticoid.

8. Generally, there appears to be a relationship between a lower intake of fat and reduced risk of cancers. It is possible that it is a higher intake of fruits and vegetables that provides the protective factor. The tie between NIDDM and hypertension and fat intake is indirect. Both disorders stress the circulatory system. The additional effects of a high fat dietary intake on the circulatory system may increase this negative the effect. For these disorders, excessive weight may be an initiating factor. Overconsumption of fats may further exacerbate excessive weight.

Types of Fatty Acids
1. single bonded carbon chains
2. one unsaturated double bonds
3. shortening
4. dairy products
5. palm
6. coconut
7. olive
8. canola
9. corn
10. fish
11. ↑ blood cholesterol
12. ↓ blood cholesterol

Triglyceride Digestion
1. foods broken into smaller pieces
2. peristalsis
3. gastric lipase
4. hydrolyzed
5. triglycerides
6. fatty acids
7. monoglycerides
8. glycerol

Practice Exam
1. D	3. D	5. D	7. A	9. C
2. C	4. A	6. C	8. D	10. D

NCLEX Questions
1. B	2. E	3. C	4. E

Chapter 6 PROTEIN

"Protein in food is our only source of amino acids, which are absolutely necessary to make the thousands of proteins that form every aspect of the human body."

IMPORTANT TERMS

Write the terms from the list on the right in the correct blanks on the left.

amino acids

aminopeptidase

carboxypeptidase

chymotrypsin

deamination

denatured

dipeptidase

pepsin

proteases

protein

trypsin

urea

1. _____ organic compounds formed from chains of amino acids

2. _____ organic compounds containing carbon, hydrogen, oxygen, and nitrogen

3. _____ a change in the shape of protein structures due to heat, light, acids, or alcohol

4. _____ protein enzymes

5. _____ the gastric protease

6. _____ the primary pancreatic protease

7. _____ a pancreatic protease that hydrolyzes polypeptides into dipeptides

8. _____ a pancreatic protease that hydrolyzes polypeptides and dipeptides into amino acids

9. _____ a process through which an amino acid group breaks off from an amino acid molecule resulting in molecules of ammonia and keto acid

10. _____ product of ammonia conversion produced during deanimation

11. _____ an intestinal peptidase that releases free amino acids from amino end of short chain peptides

12. _____ an intestinal peptidase that completes the hydrolysis of proteins to amino acids

APPLIED CONTENT KNOWLEDGE

"The healthiest approach is to eat mixed sources of protein - animal and plant sources."

Karen and her husband, Roger, want to reduce their intake of fat and increase their fiber intake. Both grew up in families that prided themselves as being the "meat and potatoes" types. Suggest three strategies they could adopt to restructure their dinner plates.

QUICK REVIEW

"Amino acids, like glucose, are organic compounds made of carbon, hydrogen, and oxygen. However, amino acids also contain nitrogen, which clearly distinguishes protein from other nutrients."

1.   Describe the structure of proteins.

2.   Differentiate between essential and nonessential amino acids.

3.   List four functions of protein in the body.

4.   Describe the difference between complete protein and incomplete protein. Discuss the concept of complementary proteins.

5.   Distinguish between protein energy malnutrition, marasmus, and kwashiorkor.

Protein RDA

"The RDA for protein provides for sufficient intake of the essential amino acids and enough total protein to provide the amino groups needed to build new NEAAs."

List 3 other factors and describe their effect on the RDA for protein.

Factor: Effect:
1.   1.

2.   2.

3.   3.

54

Measures of Food Protein

"Many foods contain protein; however, the value of specific foods as protein sources varies."

Match these phrases with their correct location in the chart on the next page.

     A. -- based on weight gain when fed set amount of protein

     B. -- based on availability of protein foods to human body; highest reference protein: value of an egg is 100

     C. -- measures nitrogen digested, absorbed, and excreted by humans

     D. -- measures physiological value of food protein by rats

Method	Measures	Basis
biological value	1_____	2_____
protein efficiency ratio (PER)	3_____	4_____

Malnutrition

"Malnutrition is often caused by a number of factors affecting food availability. Although poverty tends to be a dominant influence, other forces also affect the development of malnutrition."

Identify 2 factors for each category below:

Biological
1.

2.

Social
1.

2.

Economic
1.

2.

Environmental
1.

2.

Digestion and Absorption

"During digestion, food protein is broken down to amino acids. Once absorbed, the amino acids circulate in the blood to build new proteins. "

Match these digestive and absorption actions and terms with their correct location.

amino acids	hydrochloric acid	peristalsis
aminopeptidase	pancreatic	polypeptides
dipeptides	pepsinogen	smaller food pieces mixing with saliva

Organ	Mechanical	Chemical
Mouth	1._____	none
Stomach	2._____	3._____ activated to pepsin by
		4._____ creating smaller
		5._____
Small intestine	peristalsis	polypeptides hydrolyzed by
		6._____ and intestinal
		proteases to 7._____ and
		amino acids; peptides hydrolyzed by
		8._____ and dipeptidase to
		9._____

56

Nitrogen Balance

"Nitrogen-balance studies are used to determine the protein requirements of the body throughout the life cycle and to assign value to protein quality of foods determining biological value."

Match these terms with the correct location below. Terms may be used more than once.

dietary protein sources	growth	N equilibrium	protein
eating disorders	healing	negative N balance	retained
excreted	input	nitrogen	zero N balance
extreme stress	life span	nitrogen-balance studies	
feces and urine	muscles and organs	nitrogen leaving the body	

The protein requirement of the body through the 1._____ can be assessed

through 2._____. These studies can also be used to assess 3._____quality of

foods. The body's use of protein can be determined by comparing the amount of 4._____

entering the body in food protein with the nitrogen lost from the body in 5._____.

If the amount of nitrogen consumed in foods equals the amount excreted, a person is

in 6._____ or 7._____. Healthy adults experience this when the nitrogen

8._____ (food protein) to the body equals the output (9._____).

When more nitrogen is 10._____ in the body than 11._____, positive N

balance occurs. The nitrogen 12._____ is used to form new cells for 13._____

in growing children and pregnant women. 14._____ from illness or injury may also

result in positive N balance.

When there is a breakdown of body proteins such as those of 15._____,

16._____ occurs. This means that more 17._____ is excreted from the body

than retained from dietary protein sources. Physical illness, 18._____, aging,

19._____, or starvation may result in 20._____.

PRACTICE EXAM

1. Nonessential amino acids (NEAAs):
    A. are incomplete proteins.
    B. are extra essential amino acids.
    C. are not needed from dietary intake.
    D. are not necessary for good health.

2. The amino acid pool contains _____ for protein synthesis.
    A. only essential amino acids
    B. only NEAAs
    C. contains essential and nonessential amino acids
    D. just the amino acids needed to make certain proteins

3. Functions of proteins do not include:
    A. collagen formation.
    B. component of hormones such as insulin.
    C. water balance within the body.
    D. provides essential fatty acids.

4. Antibodies, necessary for immune system functioning, are:
    A. carbohydrates.
    B. proteins.
    C. lipids.
    D. enzymes.

5. Which of the following combinations does not provide a complementary protein combination?
    A. peanut butter and jelly sandwich
    B. rice and beans with tortillas
    C. split pea soup with carrot sticks
    D. bean chili with cornbread

6. If a patient has a prolonged high fever, the effect on the body may be:
    A. denaturing of body proteins that can affect organ functioning.
    B. indicates a bacterial function that must be treated with antibiotics.
    C. has minimal effects if dietary protein intake is sufficient.
    D. is dangerous only if dietary protein intake is insufficient.

7. The RDA for protein is _____; most Americans eat _____ than this every day.
    A. 20.8 g/kg; more
    B. 10.8 g/kg; more
    C. 0.8 g/kg; less
    D. 0.8 g/kg; more

8. Vegetarian dietary patterns provide sufficient amounts of protein by combining:
   A. vegetables and fruits.
   B. legumes and grains.
   C. legumes and vegetables.
   D. grains and fruits.

9. Chemical digestion of protein takes place in the:
   A. stomach and small intestine.
   B. mouth and stomach.
   C. mouth and small intestine.
   D. stomach and large intestine.

10. An individual experiencing the eating disorder of anorexia nervosa may be in
    _____ balance.
    A. positive N balance
    B. N equilibrium
    C. negative N balance
    D. none of the above

NCLEX Questions

1. During pregnancy, women require: (PN)
   A. the same amount of protein as non-pregnant women.
   B. 20% higher intake of protein for fetus growth and needs of their own bodies.
   C. 50% higher intake of protein for fetus growth and needs of their own bodies.
   D. the same amount of protein as athletes of the same age.

2. Hospital malnutrition is not caused by: (SE)
   A. not consuming an adequate quantity of food.
   B. decreased nutrient absorption from the effects of medications.
   C. an hospital patient consuming an imbalance of lipids.
   D. side effects of illness.

3. Advantages of vegetarian dietary patterns include all of the following except:(HP)
   A. usually lower consumption of total dietary fat and cholesterol intake.
   B. higher fiber intake.
   C. tendency to result in lower body weight.
   D. particularly high levels of vitamin D within the vegan dietary pattern.

4. Social factors increasing the risk of malnutrition include all of the following(PsN)
   except:
   A. alcoholism.
   B. drug abuse.
   C. illnesses that reduce nutrient absorption.
   D. child abuse and neglect.

ANSWERS

Important Terms

1. protein
2. amino acids
3. denatured
4. proteases
5. pepsin
6. trypsin
7. chymotrypsin
8. carboxypeptidase
9. deanimation
10. urea
11. aminopeptidase
12. dipeptidase

Applied Content Knowledge

Three strategies are: 1) reduce protein servings to about 3 oz. by serving portions that are the size of a deck of cards or the size of the palm of their hands; 2) adopt 5 a Day of eating 5 fruits and vegetables a day; and 3) use sources of protein (plant and animal) from several of the Food Guide Pyramid categories.

Quick Review

1. Proteins are composed of amino acids linked in peptide chains. Amino acids contain carbon, hydrogen, oxygen, and nitrogen. Four structural levels (primary, secondary, tertiary, and quaternary) affect protein functions. The primary level is based on the number, assortment, and sequence of amino acids in the peptide chains. The secondary level affects the shape of the chain of amino acids that may be straight, folded, or coiled. When the peptide chain coils on to itself, bonding occurs that creates the tertiary structure. The quaternary level occurs when proteins contain more than one chain.

2. To form all necessary proteins, a total of 20 amino acids are required by plants and animals. The liver can create 11 of the amino acids if the components of carbon, hydrogen, oxygen, and nitrogen are available; these amino acids are nonessential amino acids (NEAAs). The other 9 are essential amino acids and must be consume through dietary intake.

3. Four functions of protein include: 1) required for growth and maintenance because tissue, muscles, and bone depend on protein structures; 2) supports transportation of nutrients as protein acts as pumps moving nutrients in and out of cells; 3) components of immune system as antibodies (proteins) defend the body from foreign virus and bacteria; and 4) maintains fluid balance between intracellular, extracellular, and interstitial compartments.

4. A complete protein contains all 9 essential amino acids in amounts that most supports protein synthesis; incomplete protein lacks one or more of the essential amino acids. By combining certain incomplete proteins, all 9 essential amino acids are provided. This process allows the proteins to "complement" each other. Combining legumes and grains provides this complementation.

5. Protein energy malnutrition (PEM) is a condition that includes malnutrition caused by a lack of protein, energy, or both. Marasmus is malnutrition caused by a lack of energy intake, while kwashiorkor is caused by a lack of protein while eating adequate energy. Each condition has different effects on the body that may necessitate different treatments. But the differences will overlap because of the multiple deficiencies that occur with any form of malnutrition.

Protein RDA

Factor:	Effect:
1. age	1. During childhood periods of growth, an increase of dietary protein is needed for muscle and tissue formation.
2. gender	2. Males have more lean body mass than women. Lean body mass requires more protein than body fat.
3. physiological state	3. Different physiological states require additional protein. During pregnancy, protein needs increase to meet the growth requirements of the fetus. Lactation necessitates extra dietary protein for formation of breast milk.

Measures of Food Protein
1. measures nitrogen digested , absorbed, and excreted by humans
2. based on availability of protein foods to human body; highest reference protein: value of an egg is 100
3. measures physiological value of food protein by rats
4. based on weight gain when fed set amount of protein

Malnutrition
Biological:
1. lack of food
2. malnutrition before or during pregnancy

Social:
1. child abuse or neglect
2. eating disorders

Economic:
1. poverty
2. under employment

Environmental:
1. famine
2. polluted water

Digestion and Absorption
1. smaller food pieces mixing with saliva
2. peristalsis
3. pepsinogen
4. hydrochloric acid(HCL)
5. polypeptides
6. pancreatic
7. dipeptides
8. aminopeptidase
9. amino acids

Nitrogen Balance
1. life span
2. nitrogen-balance studies
3. protein
4. nitrogen
5. feces and urine
6. N equilibrium
7. zero N balance
8. input
9. nitrogen leaving the body
10. retained
11. excreted
12. retained
13. growth
14. healing
15. muscles and organs
16. negative N balance
17. nitrogen
18. extreme stress
19. eating disorders
20. negative N balance

Practice Exam
1. C
2. C
3. D
4. B
5. C
6. A
7. D
8. B
9. A
10. C

NCLEX Questions
1. B
2. C
3. D
4. C

Chapter 7 VITAMINS

"Vitamins are organic molecules that are required in very small amounts."

IMPORTANT TERMS

Write the terms from the list on the left in the correct blanks on the right.

antioxidant

cheilosis

glossitis

intrinsic factor

keratomalacia

pernicious anemia

phytochemicals

spina bifida

vitamin

xerophthalmia

1._____ essential organic molecules needed in very small amounts for cellular metabolism

2._____ nonnutritive substances in plant-based foods that appear to have disease-fighting properties

3._____ inflammation of the mucous membrane of the mouth and lips (angular stomatitis) caused by riboflavin and other B vitamin deficiencies

4._____ inflammation of the tongue

5._____ a congenital defect of the spinal column causing the spinal cord to be unprotected resulting in a range of disabilities including paralysis and incontinence

6._____ a substance produced by stomach mucosa that is required for vitamin B12 absorption

7._____ inadequate red blood cell formation caused by a lack of intrinsic factor in the stomach with which to absorb vitamin B12

8._____ a compound that guards other compounds from damaging oxidation.

9._____ a condition caused by vitamin A deficiency ranging from night blindness to keratomalacia; may result in complete blindness

10._____ a condition caused by vitamin A deficiency in which the cornea becomes dry and thickens from the formation of hard protein tissue

APPLYING CONTENT KNOWLEDGE

"Vitamins are in almost all foods, yet no one food group is a good source of all vitamins."

Mark Smith, a three-year old, is having his yearly health check-up. His mom, rather proudly, tells you that Mark eats one apple and carrot sticks every day. She says that means that he gets all the vitamins he needs. How do you respond?

QUICK REVIEW

"Although vitamin deficiencies are no longer common among Americans, subgroups are at risk."

1. List the major functions and deficiency symptoms for each water-soluble vitamin.

2. List the major functions and deficiency symptoms for each fat-soluble vitamin.

3. Discuss two subgroups of Americans who are most at risk for vitamin deficiencies.

Differences of Water-soluble and Fat-soluble Vitamins

"Vitamins are divided into two categories based on their solubility in solutions."

Fill in the blanks with these terms:

bloodstream	lymphatic system	stable	unstable
excreted	possible	stored	very possible

Characteristic of:	Water-soluble Vitamins	Fat-soluble Vitamins
After absorption travels through	a._____	b._____
Excess is	c._____	d._____
During cooking tends to be	e._____	f._____
Risk of toxicity, particularly from improper use of supplements	g._____	h._____

64

Functions of Water-soluble Vitamins

"As an antioxidant, vitamin C protects folate, vitamin E , and polyunsaturated substances from destruction by oxygen as they move throughout the body."

Match these water-soluble vitamins with their functions:

biotin	niacin	riboflavin
cobalamin (B12)	pantothenic acid	thiamin
folate	pyridoxine (B6)	vitamin C

1._____, _____,_____, and_____ have roles in

energy metabolism.

2._____ functions as metabolic coenzyme affecting the synthesis of

amino acid, heme , DNA, and RNA. Fetal neural tube formation is also

dependent on _____.

3._____ is required for transport and storage of folate. It also has a

role in metabolism of fatty acids and amino acids.

4._____ is needed for metabolism of protein, carbohydrate, and fat.

5._____ is part of coenzyme A.

6._____ has many functions including as an antioxidant, coenzyme,

collagen formation and iron absorption.

Clinical Issues of Water-soluble Vitamins

"Deficiency (of folate) may result from any condition that requires cell division to speed up , including infection, cancer, burns, blood loss, GI damage, and pregnancy."

Using the terms provided, complete these statements.

alcoholism	drugs	nausea	supplements
altered nerve function	gingivitis	niacin	toxic
antibiotics	glossitis	pellagra	vitamin C
ariboflavinosis	insufficient	perncicous anemia	Wernicke-Korsakoff
beriberi	kidney stones	protein	syndrome
coenzyme A	liver damage	raw eggs	wet beriberi
diarrhea	megablastic anemia	sensory neuropathy	wound healing

Thiamin deficiency may result in 1._____ that may be categorized as dry or 2._____. 3._____ may result in a specific form of thiamin deficiency called 4._____ that requires specific clinical responses.

5._____ with cheilosis, 6._____, and dermatitis occurs if dietary intake of riboflavin is deficient.

7._____ deficiency occurs when dietary intake of niacin and 8._____ are too low; this causes the disorder of 9._____ noted by the 3 Ds (10._____, dermatitis, and dementia). In contrast, chronic intake of high-doses of 11._____ produces 12._____ symptoms of vasodilation, 13._____, gout, and arthritic reaction.

Pyridoxine deficiencies can result in dermatitis, 14._____ and anemia. Taking supplements in high doses can result in toxic effects of ataxia and 15._____.

Many 16._____ affect the use of folate in our bodies. If the effects reduce the availability of folate or if dietary intake is 17._____, 18._____ may result. During pregnancy, a deficiency may cause spina bifida or anencephaly.

19._____ and damage to the central nervous system may occur if intake of cobalamin (B12) is deficient.

Although rare, a deficiency of biotin may result from intake of avidin from 20._____ and/or long-term treatment with 21._____.

A deficiency of pantothenic acid is not possible since it is part of 22._____.

A deficiency of 23._____ leads to the disorder of scurvy. Marginal deficiencies may cause 24._____, poor 25._____, or increased risk of infection. Excess vitamin C from supplements may lead to toxic effects of cramps, 26._____, 27._____, and gout.

Food Sources Water-soluble Vitamins

"Vitamin C (in foods) is destroyed by air, light, and heat."

Match these terms with their correct location in the table:

animal   broccoli   grains   leafy green   pork   vegetables

ascorbic   cereals   intestinal   milk/dairy   poultry   whole
                                                                            widespread

Vitamin		Food Sources
thiamin		lean 1.____, whole or enriched 2.____ and flours, legumes
riboflavin		3.____ products, meat, poultry, and fish, eggs, green leafy vegetables, 4.____ and enriched grains and cereals
niacin		meats, poultry, and fish, legumes, whole and enriched 5.____, milk
pyridoxine		whole grains and cereals, legumes, 6.____, fish, pork and eggs
folate		7.____ vegetables, legumes, and 8.____ containing foods
cobalamin		9.____ foods
biotin		liver, kidneys, peanut butter, egg yolks, 10.____ synthesis
pantothenic acid		11.____ in foods
vitamin C		fruits and 12.____ (citrus fruits, tomatoes, peppers, strawberries, 13.____)

Functions of Fat-soluble Vitamins

"With sufficient exposure to ultraviolet light or sunshine, the body can manufacture its own supply of vitamin D by converting a form of cholesterol in the skin."

Complete the following sentences with these terms:

absorption	clotting	selenium
alpha-tocopherol	deposition	vitamin A
bone growth	epithelial tissues	vitamin K

Vitamin A functions to maintain 1._____ and is needed for rhodopsin formation for vision. Additional functions includes 2._____ and a role in reproduction.

Calcium and phosphorus 3._____ are dependent on sufficient vitamin D. Once absorbed these and other minerals require vitamin D for 4._____ in bones.

Vitamin E or 5._____ is an antioxidant protecting polyunsaturated fatty acids (PUFA) and 6._____. It also has other antioxidant functions in a system with 7._____ and ascorbic acid.

8._____ acts as a cofactor in synthesis of blood 9._____ factors and has a role in protein formation.

Clinical Issues of Fat-soluble Vitamins

"Premature infants and newborns are unable to immediately produce vitamin K; their guts are too sterile, free from the microflora necessary to produce vitamin K.. Hospitals in the United States routinely give newborns an intramuscular dose of vitamin K to prevent hemorrhagic disease."

Complete these short answer questions.

A. Deficiencies of fat-soluble vitamins may be caused by primary or secondary deficiencies.

   A primary deficiency is caused by:

   A secondary deficiency may be caused by:

B. Vitamin A deficiency results in effects reacted to its function in the body.
   How are the eyes affected by vitamin A deficiency?

   Toxic effects cause hypervitaminosis A that is associated with supplement intake.
   Describe the symptoms associate with hypervitaminosis A.

C. Vitamin D deficiency affects bone formation.
   What are the two disorders that may result?

   A chronic excessive intake, particularly from supplements, may cause?

D. Vitamin E deficiency is rare but may occur because of malabsorption resulting in neurological disorders. What kind of deficiency would that be?

E. Blood coagulation is inhibited by vitamin K deficiency. The deficiency may be caused by a malabsorption disorder or drug/medication interactions. Long term antibiotic use may adversely affect vitamin K levels in the body. How?

Food Sources of Fat-soluble Vitamins

"If we consume more than the daily requirement of a fat-soluble vitamin, our bodies store the excess rather excreting it."

Match these terms with their correct location in the table:

body synthesis   milk   vegetable oil   whole grains

intestinal synthesis   orange   vegetables

Vitamin	Food Sources
vitamin A	deep green, yellow, and 1._____ fruits and 2._____; whole and fortified 3._____; liver
vitamin D	animal (fat) sources; 4._____
vitamin E	5._____, 6._____, seeds, nuts, green leafy vegetables
vitamin K	green leafy vegetables; 7._____

PRACTICE EXAM

1.   Thiamin, riboflavin, and niacin function as:
      A. antioxidants
      B. phytochemicals
      C. coenzymes in energy metabolism
      D. hormones

2.   An individual who chronically ingests excessive amounts of alcohol may be at
      risk for thiamin deficiency because:
      A. decreased food intake
      B. reduced intestinal absorption
      C. additional use of thiamin by the liver to detoxify alcohol
      D. all of the above

3.   In the American diet, a major source of riboflavin is:
      A. milk and other dairy products
      B. fruits, particularly citrus fruits
      C. vegetables, especially cruciferous fruits
      D. green leafy vegetables including iceberg lettuce

4.   A precursor of niacin is _____; this means that a diet containing enough
      _____ will provide sufficient amounts of niacin.
      A. tryptophan; protein
      B. fiber; complex carbohydrates
      C. fatty acids; lipids
      D. lecithin; phospholipids

5.   A number of drugs may affect the bioavailability and metabolism of vitamin B6.
      The most commonly used of these drugs is:
      A. antibiotics
      B. aspirin
      C. oral contraceptive agents
      D. antihistamines

6.   In order for folate to be used by the body, _____ must be available.
      Therefore before a deficiency of folate is treated, a deficiency of _____
      must be considered.
      A. niacin; tryptophan
      B. cobalamin (B12); cobalamin (B12)
      C. cobalamin (B12); ascorbic acid
      D. beta carotene; vitamin A

7. Biotin is available by:
    A. intestinal synthesis by bacterial microorganism
    B. exposure of the skin to the sun
    C. the precursor beta carotene
    D. the precursor tryptophan

8. To consume enough pantothenic acid, individuals must:
    A. carefully plan their diets to include food sources of pantothenic acid
    B. eat lots of fruits and vegetables that are the only source
    C. simply eat foods; pantothenic acid is widespread in foods
    D. take supplements to be sure of adequate intake

9. Vitamin C is lacking from which of the following meals?
    A. hamburger with carrot and celery sticks and a diet cola
    B. hamburger with lettuce and tomato and a glass of milk
    C. pasta primavera (tomatoes, peppers, onions, and broccoli) and a glass of wine
    D. garlic chicken, roasted potatoes and a citrus fruit salad

10. An early sign of vitamin A deficiency is:
    A. bleeding gums
    B. night blindness
    C. blindness
    D. anemia

NCLEX Questions

1. Vitamin K is: (PN)
    A. a cofactor for blood clotting
    B. a factor for rhodopsin formation
    C. antioxidant with selenium and ascorbic acid
    D. A and B
    E. A and C

2. Factors that may precipitate the development of rickets include: (SE)
    A. possible lack of dietary sources if vegetarian
    B. living in a geographical region with limited sunlight exposure
    C. darker skin pigmentation combined with concealing clothing
    D. all of the above

3. As our dietary intake of _____ increases, so does our need for _____.   (HP)
    Fortunately, _____ are food sources of _____.
    A. protein; vitamin D; meat, fish and poultry; vitamin D
    B. lipids; vitamin A; butter and butterfat; vitamin A
    C. polyunsaturated fats; vitamin E; vegetable oils containing PUFAs; vitamin E
    D. carbohydrates; vitamin E; refined grains; vitamin E

4. A 25 year-old female employee approaches the nurse at the corporate   (PsN)
    health center about a health concern. She would like to receive a shot of vitamin
    B12 because she's been feeling tired lately. Her grandmother recently got a shot
    and now feels much better. How should the nurse advise her?
    A. explain that the elderly may have trouble absorbing vitamin B12 which is why
        her grandmother felt better
    B. it is unusual for a young person to be deficient in vitamin B12 unless a vegan
        dietary pattern is followed
    C. review her daily activities and sleep habits to assess other sources of fatigue
        and if none are apparent suggest a complete physical examination with the
        primary care provider
    D. A and B
    E. A, B, and C

ANSWERS
Important Terms
1. vitamin	3. cheilosis	5. spina bifida	7. pernicious anemia	9. xerophthalmia
2. phytochemicals	4. glossitis	6. intrinsic factors	8. antioxidant	10. keratomalacia

Applying Content Knowledge

Although an apple and carrot sticks are good sources of vitamins they do not provide all the essential vitamins. We also need to eat foods from the other food groups in addition to fruits and vegetables to be assured of eating adequate amounts of vitamins.

Quick Review

1. Refer to Table 7-3 (page 165) for a list of the functions and deficiency symptoms of water-soluble vitamins.

2. Refer to Table 7-6 (page 174) for a list of the functions and deficiency symptoms of fat-soluble vitamins.

3. Two subgroups of Americans who are most at risk for vitamin deficiencies are the elderly and individuals who chronically consume excess amounts of alcohol. The elderly are at risk because of difficulties with buying, preparing, and even chewing foods that are the best sources of vitamins. Individuals with alcohol consumption problems are at risk because of inadequate dietary intake, increased requirement for thiamin to detoxify the alcohol and decreased absorption of nutrients from the effect of alcohol on the gastrointestinal tract.

Differences of Water-soluble and Fat-soluble Vitamins
a. bloodstream	c. excreted	e. unstable	g. possible
b. lymphatic system	d. stored	f. stable	h. very possible

Functions of Water-soluble Vitamins
1. thiamin, riboflavin, niacin, pyridoxine (B6)	4. biotin
2. folate; folate	5. pantothenic acid
3. cobalamin (B12)	6. vitamin C

Clinical Issues of Water-soluble Vitamins
1. beriberi	10. diarrhea	19. pernicious anemia
2. wet beriberi	11. supplements	20. raw eggs
3. alcoholism	12. toxic	21. antibiotics
4. Wernicke-Korsakoff syndrome	13. liver damage	22. coenzyme A
5. ariboflavinosis	14. altered nerve function	23. vitamin C
6. glossitis	15. sensory neuropathy	24. gingivitis
7. niacin	16. drugs	25. wound healing
8. protein	17. insufficient	26. nausea
9. pellagra	18. megablastic anemia	27. kidney stones

Food Sources Water-soluble Vitamins
1. pork	3. milk/dairy	5. cereals/grains	7. leafy green	9. animal	11. widespread
2. grains	4. whole	6. poultry	8. ascorbic	10. intestinal	12. vegetables
					13. broccoli

Functions of Fat-soluble Vitamins

1. epithelial tissues	4. deposition	7. selenium
2. bone growth	5. alpha-tocopherol	8. vitamin K
3. mineralization	6. vitamin A	9. clotting

Clinical Issues of Fat-soluble Vitamins

A. A primary deficiency is caused by a lack of the vitamin in the foods that are eaten. A secondary deficiency may be caused by malabsorption of fats or drug/nutrient interactions.

B. The effects on eyes progresses as a vitamin A deficiency increases. First night blindness occurs leading to hardening of cornea that eventually causes permanent blindness.

Symptoms of hypervitaminosis includes nausea, blistered skin, vomiting, and enlarged liver and spleen.

C. The two disorders are rickets and osteomalacia. Chronic excessive intake of vitamin D may cause hypercalcemia and hypercalciuria.

D. A secondary deficiency is caused by malabsorption.

E. The antibiotics may kill the intestinal micro flora that provides some of the vitamin K used by the body.

Food Sources of Fat-soluble Vitamins

1. orange	3. milk	5. vegetable oil	7. intestinal synthesis
2. vegetable	4. body synthesis	6. whole grains	

Practice Exam

1. C	3. A	5. C	7. A	9. A
2. D	4. A	6. B	8. C	10. B

NCLEX Questions

1. A	2. D	3. C	4. E

Chapter 8 WATER AND MINERALS

"An ever-circulating ocean of fluid bathes all the cells of our bodies; this fluid allows for chemical reactions, transmission of nerve impulses, and transportation of nutrients and waste products throughout the body."

IMPORTANT TERMS

Write the terms from this list in the correct blanks below.

aldosterone

antidiuretic hormone (ADH)

calcitonin

calcitriol

heme iron

insensible perspiration

nonheme iron

osteoporosis

parathormone

pica

1. _____ water lost invisibly through evaporation from the lungs and skin

2. _____ a hormone secreted by the pituitary gland in response to low fluid levels; affects kidneys to decrease excretion of water

3. _____ a hormone secreted by the adrenal gland in response to sodium levels in kidneys; affects kidneys to balance fluid levels as needed

4. _____ a hormone that raises blood calcium levels; secreted by the parathyroid gland in response to low blood calcium levels

5. _____ the active vitamin D hormone that raises blood calcium levels

6. _____ a hormone that reacts in response to high blood levels of calcium; released by the Special C cells of the thyroid gland

7. _____ a multifactorial disorder in which bone density is reduced and remaining bone is brittle, breaking easily

8. _____ dietary iron found in animal foods of meat, fish, and poultry

9. _____ dietary iron found in plant foods

10. _____ a condition characterized by a hunger and appetite for non-food substances

APPLYING CONTENT KNOWLEDGE

"Although they do contain water, coffee, tea, and alcohol act as diuretics, causing an increase in water loss via the kidneys as urine."

The camp nurse gives a talk to the camp staff about the signs of fluid volume deficit. She encourages the counselors to be sure the campers drink fluids throughout the day. One counselor responds, "Oh, that's no problem. The kids guzzle flavored ice tea all day long." How should she respond?

QUICK REVIEW

"Minerals are inorganic substances composed of elements from the rock of the earth."

1.   Identify three functions of water.

2.   Describe fluid volume deficit and fluid volume excess.

3.   List three factors that may affect the bioavailability of minerals.

4.   List the primary functions, deficiency, and toxicity symptoms for the major minerals.

5.   List the primary functions, deficiency, and toxicity symptoms for the trace minerals.

Mineral Classifications

"To maintain body levels, major minerals are needed daily from dietary sources in amounts of 100 mg or higher. In contrast, trace minerals are required daily in amounts less than or equal to 20 mg."

Complete the chart below with the seven major minerals and nine trace minerals.

MAJOR MINERALS   TRACE MINERALS

1. _____   1. _____

2. _____   2. _____

3. _____   3. _____

4. _____   4. _____

5. _____   5. _____

6. _____   6. _____

7. _____   7. _____

                                  8. _____

                                  9. _____

Functions of Minerals

"Minerals serve a variety of functions in our bodies."

1. List two major minerals that perform the following functions:

    A. affect bone and tooth formation

        1.

        2.

    B. influence nerve and muscle functions

        1.

        2.

    C. maintain proper acid-base balance

        1.

        2.

    D. component of blood clotting

        1.

        2.

    E. affects blood pressure

        1.

        2.

    F. influences fluid regulation as an electrolyte

        1.

        2.

2. List trace minerals that perform the following functions:

    A. influences bone and tooth formation

        1.

    B. antioxidant functions with vitamin E

        1.

    C. role in carbohydrate metabolism (list 2 minerals)

        1.

        2.

    D. distributes oxygen in hemoglobin and myoglobin

        1.

    E. acts as a cofactor for numerous enzymes

        1.

    F. functions as a coenzyme

        1.

    G. required for thyroxin production

        1.

    H. necessary for BMR regulation

        1.

Factors of Calcium Absorption

"Our bodies absorb calcium based on physiological need."

Place these factors of calcium absorption in the appropriate column:

binders

certain medications

dietary fat

digestive mass acidity

high fiber intake

lactose

laxatives

physiological need

phytic acid and oxalic acid

regular weight-bearing exercise

sedentary lifestyle

sufficient vitamin D

INCREASES ABSORPTION:

1._____

2._____

3._____

4._____

5._____

DECREASES ABSORPTION:

6._____

7._____

8._____

9._____

10._____

11._____

12._____

Osteoporosis and Bone Density

"In contrast to osteomalacia, osteoporosis is multifactorial and all the factors are tied to bone mineral density."

List two factors that affect bone density but cannot be modified. Describe their affect on bone density.

Factor: Affect on bone density:

1. _____   _____

2. _____   _____

List two lifestyle factors that affect bone density. Describe their influence on bone density.

Factor: Influence on bone density:

3. _____   _____

4. _____   _____

Iron

"Iron deficiency has been a public health problem for many years."

The chart below contains factors that affect iron absorption and factors that increase the risk of iron deficiency. Use the following terms to complete the chart:

antacids   coffee and tea   menses   plant food
binders   dietary iron   pagophagia   poultry
chronic   internal bleeding   pica   skillet
                                                                        vitamin C

EFFECT	FACTORS
ABSORPTION INCREASED by	- eating iron-containing foods with foods that contain (1.)_____ such as orange juice or melon - eating meat, fish, or (2.)_____ foods - eating plant and animal sources of (3.)_____ at the same time - using cast iron (4.)_____ to cook acidic foods
ABSORPTION DECREASED by	- drinking (5.)_____ with iron-containing foods - high-fiber meals that contain (6.)_____ with (7.)_____ such as oxalates and phytates - (8.)_____ - chronic use of (9.)_____ - excessive intake of other minerals
DEFICIENCY RISK INCREASED by	- lack of sufficient intake of iron-rich food - (10.)_____ weight loss dieting - loss of blood from (11.)_____ for females of childbearing ages - loss of blood from (12.)_____ in the GI tract such as from ulcers or hemorrhoids - practice of pica, geophagia, amylophagia, and/or (13.)_____

PRACTICE EXAM

1.   Functions of water include all of the following except:
      A. transports nutrients and waste products
      B. provides shape and rigidity to cells
      C. acts as an antioxidants
      D. acts as lubricant

2.   The body uses calcium for:
      A. central nervous system functioning
      B. blood clotting
      C. blood pressure regulation
      D. all of the above

3.   Sources of phosphorus are:
      A. difficult to find
      B. widespread in foods
      C. may often include supplements if a person is lactose intolerant
      D. must be carefully added to dietary intake plans

4.   An unexpected source of magnesium may be:
      A. processed foods
      B. soft water
      C. hard water
      D. alcohol

5.   Sulfur is a component of:
      A. protein structures
      B. adipose tissues
      C. carbohydrates
      D. A and B

6.   Electrolytes include:
      A. potassium
      B. phosphorus
      C. sodium
      D. A and C plus chloride
      E. B and C plus chloride

7.   _____ is the major extracellular electrolyte while _____ is the major intracellular electrolyte.
      A. calcium; potassium
      B. sodium; chloride
      C. sodium; potassium
      D. potassium; sodium

8. Most common sources of sodium in the American diet include:
    A. sodium supplements
    B. processed foods and salt added when cooking
    C. in foods naturally
    D. A and B
    E. B and C

9. The gastric juice hydrochloric acid is produced by the _____. It contains the mineral _____.
    A. stomach; chloride
    B. small intestine; chloride
    C. stomach; sodium
    D. small intestine; sodium

10. Individuals at risk for zinc deficiency may include:
    A. older persons with inadequate dietary intake
    B. children with picky eating styles
    C. teenage males
    D. A and B
    E. B and C

11. Too much fluoride causes fluorosis. Symptoms include:
    A. brown spotted teeth
    B. pitted teeth
    C. excessive decay
    D. A and B

12. Selenium is:
    A. is often recommended in megadoses for its antioxidant function
    B. safe at any level of food or supplement intake
    C. very toxic at five times the RDA and may cause severe liver damage
    D. a nutrient for which consuming the RDA is difficult

13. Toxicity from copper may occur from:
    A. supplements
    B. eating too many servings of green leafy vegetables
    C. A and B
    D. none of the above

NCLEX Questions

1. Water makes up _____ of the weight of an average adult and _____ (PN)
    for infants.
    A. 50-65%; 50-65%
    B. 50-65%; 75%
    C. 75%; 50%
    D. 95%; 50-65%

2. If a client is taking a potassium wasting diuretic, which of the following foods
    should not be suggested as a source of potassium?   (SE)
    A. dairy products
    B. oranges
    C. bananas
    D. processed convenience foods

3. Iodine deficiency results in _____, but fortification of _____ (HP)
    has reduced the incidence of this condition in the U.S.
    A. pica; flour
    B. goiter; salt
    C. goiter; flour
    D. hemosiderosis; salt

4. Individuals with chronic excessive alcohol consumption and persons who   (PsN)
    are genetically at risk for _____ may experience symptoms of iron
    overload. These symptoms may include _____.
    A. pica; increased wound healing
    B. hemochromatosis; increased body strength
    C. hemochromatosis; liver and heart damage
    D. hydroxyapatite; liver and heart damage

ANSWERS

Important Terms

1. insensible perspiration   3. aldosterone   5. calcitriol   7. osteoporosis   9. nonheme iron

2. antidiuretic hormone   4. parathormone 6. calcitonin   8. heme iron   10. pica

Applying Content Knowledge

        The camp nurse can explain that although the flavored ice tea contains water, it also contains caffeine. The caffeine acts as a diuretic causing fluid loss; this means that beverages containing caffeine (including sodas containing caffeine) cannot be counted towards fluid intake to maintain proper hydration. The campers can drink plain water or fruit juices to meet their fluid requirements.

Quick Review

1. Three functions of water include: regulates body temperature; acts as a solvent; and provides shape and rigidity to cells.

2. Fluid volume deficit (FVD) occurs when the fluid levels in the body are very low. This includes vascular, cellular, intracellular dehydration. It may occur from diarrhea, vomiting, a high fever, or excessive perspiration. Symptoms may include decreased urination, dry mouth, and unusual sleepiness.
     Fluid volume excess (FVE) occurs when a higher than normal amount of fluid is retained causing edema. It may be due to excess fluid intake, excess sodium intake or impaired fluid regulatory mechanism. Most often edema passes as the sodium content of the body rebalances but in some individuals, hypertension may occur.

3. Three factors that may affect the bioavailability of minerals are binders, the source of the minerals, and food processing. The presence of binders in plant foods may result in indigestible compounds causing minerals to be excreted without being absorbed. Minerals from animal foods are more bioavailable than minerals found in plant foods. Food processing may cause the loss of minerals during refining processes and these minerals are often not returned to the final food product.

4. Refer to Table 8-6 (page 197) in the text to review the primary function, deficiency, and toxicity symptoms of major minerals.

5. Refer to Table 8-7 (page 206-207) in the text to review the primary functions, deficiency, and toxicity symptoms of trace minerals.

Mineral Classifications

Major minerals
1. calcium
2. chloride
3. magnesium
4. phosphorus
5. potassium
6. sodium
7. sulfur

Trace Minerals
1. chromium
2. copper
3. fluoride
4. iodine
5. iron
6. manganese
7. molybdenum
8. selenium
9. zinc

Functions of Minerals

1.
A. 1. calcium   2. phosphorus
B. 1. calcium   2. magnesium
C. 1. chloride   2. sodium

D. 1. calcium   2. magnesium
E. 1. calcium   2. sodium
F. 1. sodium   2. potassium

2.
A. 1. fluoride
B. 1. selenium
C. 1. zinc 2. chromium
D. 1. iron

E. 1. zinc
F. 1. copper
G. 1. iodine
H. 1. iodine

Factors of Calcium Absorption

Increases Absorption
1. digestive mass acidity
2. lactose
3. physiological need
4. regular weight-bearing exercise
5. sufficient vitamin D

Decreases Absorption
6. binders
7. certain medications
8. dietary fat
9. high fiber intake
10. laxatives
11. phytic acid and oxalic acid
12. sedentary lifestyle

Osteoporosis and Bone Density

1. gender - Males tend to naturally have greater bone density than women. When bone density slowly decreases as part of the aging process, male bones are more dense. Therefore, the density is proportionally greater than female bones. Females also experience changes in estrogen levels that can result in varying degrees of bone demineralization.

2. family history - The bone density of an individual may be influenced by genetics.

3. nutrition/calcium intake - Long-term marginal deficiencies of calcium may reduce bone density.

4. sedentary lifestyle - Lack of weight-bearing exercise decreases bone density.

Iron

1. vitamin C
2. poultry
3. dietary iron
4. skillets

5. coffee and tea
6. plant foods
7. binders
8. pica

9. antacids
10. chronic
11. menses
12. internal bleeding
13. pagophagia

Practice Exam

1. C	3. B	5. A	7. C	9. A	11. D	13. A
2. D	4. C	6. D	8. E	10. D	12. C	

NCLEX Question

1. B   2. D   3. B   4. C

Chapter 9 ENERGY AND FITNESS

"The abilities to perform work, produce change, and maintain life all require energy."

IMPORTANT TERMS

Write the terms from the list on the left in the correct blanks on the right.

adenosine triphosphate (ATP)

aerobic glycolysis

amenorrhea

anaerobic glycolysis

basal metabolism

ergogenic aids

glycolysis

oxygen debt

resting energy expenditure (REE)

thermic effect of food (TEF)

1._____ an energy-rich compound used for all energy-requiring processes in the body

2._____ the conversion of glucose to carbon compounds

3. Oxygen debt the amount of oxygen required to clear lactic acid buildup from the body

4. aerobic glycolysis the conversion of glucose to lactic acid to provide energy in the absence of oxygen

5. anaerobic glycolysis the conversion of glucose to ATP for energy when oxygen is available

6. basal metabolism the amount of energy required to maintain life-sustaining activities for a specific period of time

7._____ the energy expended in a normal life situation while at rest, and energy used following meals and exercise

8._____ an increase of cellular activity when food is eaten

9._____ lack of menstruation

10. _____ drugs and dietary regimens believed by some, but not proven, to increase strength, power, and endurance

APPLYING CONTENT KNOWLEDGE

"The energy source that muscles use during exercise depends on the intensity and length of exercise, the person's fitness level, and the foods eaten."

Darren White, a college student, just started an aerobic exercise plan to lose some "fat." Because he feels really tired, he stops by the health center of his college and chats with a nurse practitioner about his exercise program. He asks, "If my muscles use simple carbohydrates for energy, why isn't it okay for me to have a soda and a candy bar rather than a regular meal? It's all kilocalories, isn't it?" How might the nurse practitioner respond?

QUICK REVIEW

"In addition to preventing heart disease, exercise may decrease the risk of colon cancer, stroke, and hypertension."

1.   Name the three primary energy sources for the body. Briefly describe their energy pathways.

2.   Complete this table:

	Takes place in:	Oxygen required?	Energy source for:
Anaerobic Pathway	_____	_____	_____
Aerobic Pathway	_____	_____	_____

3.   Discuss the three components of fitness.

4.   Identify four chronic disorders for which regular exercise may prevent, reduce the risk, or treat the disorders.

Components of Total Energy Requirements

"Our daily energy requirement depends on many variables, including basal metabolism, physical activity, and the thermic effect of food."

Use these terms to complete the table below:

7-10 %	body fat	fasting	lean muscle
20-30 %	body size	foods	nutrients
60-75 %	cell	intensity	thyroid function
aging	dieting	larger body size	weight loss dieting

VARIABLE	AFFECTED BY	ACTIONS
basal metabolism (BMR) 1._____ of total energy	age, 2._____, body temperature, body size and lean body mass, stress of 3._____ or starvation, menstruation, 4._____	Increase BMR: 5._____ mass, being male, puberty hyperthyroidism, pregnancy Decrease BMR: 6._____, being female, sleep, hypothyroidism, 7._____, undernutrition (fasting or imposed starvation such 8._____)
physical activity 9._____ of total energy	10._____, activity level, 11._____ of movement	Increases with 12._____, greater activity levels and more intense movements
thermic effect of 13._____ 14._____ of total energy	eating	Accounts for energy to digest, absorb, metabolize, and store 15._____ from foods; increases body 16._____ activity

Health Benefits of Fitness

"An inactive person has twice the risk of developing coronary artery disease than one who exercises regularly."

List four ways that regular physical exercise reduces the risk of coronary artery disease:

1.   3.

2.   4.

Water: The Essential Ingredient

"Water is the nutrient most critical to athletic performance."

Maintenance of adequate body fluid levels is important for athletic performance in competition as well as during practice sessions. Avoidance of dehydration or fluid volume deficit (FVD) is equally important for individuals striving for physical fitness through non-competitive athletic activities.

Place these symptoms below the appropriate heading:

   A. blood volume decreases and body temperature increases
   B. clear urine throughout day
   C. confusion
   D. loss of coordination
   E. replacing each lost pound with 2 cups of fluid

               DEHYDRATION (FVD)   HYDRATION

                 _____   _____

                 _____   _____

                 _____

"The athlete's sense of thirst is not the best indicator that the body needs water; fluid needs may be greater than thirst can gauge."

Complete the sentence below using these numbers: 1, 2, 5, 10, 15, 20. Numbers may be used more than once.

To maintain adequate water intake, before, during , and after an event or practice

session, an individual should drink ___ to ___ cups of fluid ___ to ___ minutes

before exercise and ___ cup of water every ___ to ___ minutes during exercise.

PRACTICE EXAM

1. Released energy from foods are stored in a special fuel called:
    A. kilocalories.
    B. adenosine triphosphate (ATP).
    C. creatinine.
    D. glycolysis.

2. Glycolysis is the process through which glucose releases _____ and
    _____. Since it is an _____, oxygen is not needed.
    A. nicotinic acid; ATP; aerobic pathway
    B. pyruvic acid; ATP; aerobic pathway
    C. pyruvic acid; ATP; anaerobic pathway
    D. pyruvic acid; REE; anaerobic pathway

3. An _____ condition occurs when oxygen is available to the muscles.
    A. aerobic
    B. anaerobic
    C. cardiovascular
    D. lactic

4. When _____ accumulates in muscles it is due to a lack of _____ in an
    anaerobic exertion.
    A. phosphorous; oxygen
    B. lactic acid; protein
    C. lactic acid; oxygen
    D. ATP; oxygen

5. The relationship between regular aerobic physical exercise and reduced risk of heart disease is most tied to:
   A. improved cardiovascular endurance.
   B. increased muscular strength.
   C. enhanced flexibility.
   D. none of the above

6. Cyclists, swimmers and runners training for endurance events may require a higher percentage of energy from _____.
   A. protein
   B. lipids
   C. water
   D. carbohydrates

7. If college athletes consume less than the minimum kcalorie requirement of 1800 to 2000 kcalories a day, they are:
   A. at an advantage by being at an optimum minimum weight.
   B. at greater risk for iron deficiency, stress fractures, and listlessness.
   C. in danger, if female, of experiencing amenorrhea and future osteoporosis.
   D. B and C
   E. A, B, and C

8. John Gordon is an athlete who trains four days a week. He has read that athletes need more protein. Although he eats animal protein sources at most meals and drinks skim milk regularly, he has started using a protein shake twice a day. Is this shake necessary? Why or why not?
   A. The shake is not needed. Athletes do not need any more protein than sedentary individuals.
   B. The shake is not needed. Most athletes, such as John, consume sufficient amounts of protein to meet their extra needs of 1.0 to 1.5 g/kg body weight.
   C. The shake is needed. Athletes, such as John, need substantially more protein than sedentary individuals to meet additional protein needs of twice the RDA of 56 grams per day.
   D. The shake is needed. The protein in the shake provides better quality protein than the protein contained in animal sources.

NCLEX Questions
1. For optimum athletic performance, the nutritional needs of athletes are: (PN)
   A. substantially greater than nonathletes requiring the use of food and vitamin supplements.
   B. the same as nonathletes.
   C. not different from nonathletes.
   D. not different from nonathletes, with the exception of increased need for kcalories and fluids.

96

2. Carbohydrate loading is a process to achieve maximum muscle glycogen (SE) stores. It involves:
   A. combining increased fat and carbohydrate intake 30 days before a long endurance event.
   B. combining rest and increased carbohydrate intake 2 weeks before a long endurance event.
   C. combining rest and increased carbohydrate intake 3 days before a long endurance event.
   D. combining increased exercise to point of exhaustion and depleting glycogen before the event.

3. Increasing activity level and _____ are two factors for maintaining (HP) healthy body weight. The benefits of physical activity include _____, _____ and burns kcalories.
   A. consuming a low-fat diet; raises basal metabolic rate; increases lean body mass
   B. consuming a high-fat diet; lowers basal metabolic rate; decreases lean body fat
   C. consuming a low-fat diet; raises basal metabolic rate; increases body fat composition
   D. consuming a high-fat diet; lowers basal metabolic rate; increases lean body mass

4. Athletes may be so concerned about appearance that they may consume too (PsN) few calories to maintain body weight and body fat levels that are too low for good health. This may lead to:
   A. osteoporosis.
   B. iron deficiency.
   C. amenorrhea (for females).
   D. all of the above

ANSWERS

Important Terms

1. adenosine triphosphate (ATP)
2. glycolysis
3. oxygen debt
4. anaerobic glycolysis
5. aerobic glycolysis
6. basal metabolism
7. resting energy expenditure (REE)
8. thermic effect of food (TEF)
9. amenorrhea
10. ergogenic aids

Applying Content Knowledge

The body depends on protein, fat, fiber, and complex carbohydrate for optimum functioning, muscle-building, and energy levels. A candy bar and a soda provide simple carbohydrates but few other nutrients. Although an occasional candy bar and soda are acceptable, if they often replace meals, nutrient deficiencies may result that would hinder his fitness program.

Quick Review

1. The three primary energy sources are lipids, carbohydrates, and protein. The glucose pathway results in energy release as glycolysis produces pyruvic acid and ATP. If the process is incomplete then lactic acid builds up in the absence of oxygen. When the process is complete, the converted energy nutrients enter the TCA cycle as acetyl CoA. The lipid pathway occurs as triglycerides are broken down to glycerol and fatty acids and enters glycolysis. The glycerol is turned into pyruvic acid and used for energy. Fatty acids are processed into acetyl CoA entering the TCA cycle. Protein are broken down to amino acids and then deanimated. The nitrogen amino groups are converted by the liver while the other amino groups enter the energy pathways at different points.

2. a. cell cytoplasm   no   short intense exercise

   b. cell mitochondria   yes   low to moderate exercise/ endurance activities

3. The three components of fitness are flexibility, muscular strength and endurance, and cardiovascular endurance. Flexibility is being able to move muscles to their full extent without injury. Muscular strength and endurance is the ability to do prolonged work of intensive exertion. Cardiovascular endurance is the level at which the body can take in, provide and use oxygen for physical work.

4. Four chronic disorders are diabetes mellitus, hypertension, osteoporosis and coronary artery disease.

Components of Total Energy Requirements

1. 60-75%
2. sex
3. fasting
4. thyroid
5. lean muscle
6. body fat
7. aging
8. weight loss dieting
9. 20-30%
10. body size
11. intensity
12. larger body size
13. foods
14. 7-10%
15. nutrients
16. cell

Health Benefits of Fitness

1. improves cardiovascular strength
2. decreases blood pressure
3. aids in losing and/or maintaining weight
4. alters blood lipid and lipoprotein levels

Water: The Essential Ingredient

Dehydration: A, C, D   Hydration: B, E
1, 2, 5, 10, 1, 15, 20

Practice Exam

1. B
2. C
3. A
4. C
5. A
6. D
7. D
8. B

NCLEX Questions

1. D
2. C
3. A
4. D

Chapter 10 MANAGEMENT OF BODY FAT LEVELS

"Lifelong management of body fat levels provides a more holistic health approach to body size than does body weight."

IMPORTANT TERMS

Match the terms on the left with the correct definitions on the right.

adipocytes

appetite

bioelectric impedance analysis (BIA)

body image

computerized tomography (CT)

densitometry

hunger

hyperplasia

hypertrophy

management

multifactorial phenotype

visceral fat

1. _management_ the use of available resources to achieve a predetermined goal

2. _Body Image_ the perceptions we have of the physical appearance or attractiveness of our bodies

3. _hunger_ desire for food

4. _appetite_ a physiological need for food

5. _visceral fat_ fat that is within the abdominal cavity

6. _adipocytes_ cells specialized for storage of fat

7. _hyperplasia_ an increase in the number of cells occurring during the growth spurts accompanying normal development

8. _hypertrophy_ an increase in the size of cells

9. _densitometry_ underwater weighing

10. _____ an imaging technique for determining body fat composition

11. _____ a method using a very mild electric charge to estimate lean body mass in order to determine body fat composition

12. _____ a characteristic that is the product of numerous genetic and environmental factors

APPLYING CONTENT KNOWLEDGE

"In setting goals, we must consider two almost opposing factors:(1) our unique and individual values, needs, and characteristics and (2) the limits to the extent of control we have over our bodies and our level of fatness."

Carol Johnson eats a moderately low-fat diet, doesn't overeat and exercises 3 to 4 times a week. Her body fat level is about 32%. Her friend, Barbara Gordon, also eats a moderately low-fat diet, doesn't overeat and exercises 3 to 4 times a week. But compared to Carol, Barbara's body fat level is in the low range of 22%. Explain how their body fat levels could differ.

QUICK REVIEW

"From both a health and an appearance perspective, it is not only the amount of fat but its location that is important."

1.   Describe the influence of culture on body image.

2.   Explain the relationship between body fat location and health risks.

3.   Discuss the non-diet approach to management of body fat levels.
        Describe normalizing eating patterns and hunger-directed eating.

Body Fatness and Health

"Most of our evidence of the association of fatness and physical health comes from epidemiological studies."

1.   List 3 conditions for which risk is increased by higher levels of body fat, particularly in the abdominal area.

        1.   2.   3.

2.   List 3 conditions for which risk is increased by obesity but are not usually life threatening.

        1.   2.   3.

3.   List 2 conditions that are not affected by obesity.

        1.   2.

Body Fat: Essential Versus Healthy Levels

"In women, the concept of essential fat must be expanded to include gender-specific fat in their breasts, pelvic region, and buttocks that is apparently an evolutionary feature that provides energy during childbearing and lactation."

We cannot live without some body fat. Individual differences affect our levels of body fat. Body fat can be measured as a percentage of body weight. Minimum levels have been suggested to account for essential needs of body functions and levels that are considered healthy.

Use the following ranges of body fat percentage of body weight to complete the chart below:

| 3% - 8% | 12% - 14% | 20% - 22% | 25% - 30% |

	ESSENTIAL Range		HEALTHY Range
FEMALES	_____		_____
MALES	_____		_____

Body Composition and Active Lifestyles

"Although exercise is not a panacea, it is one of the few factors consistently associated with success in maintaining a healthy body composition."

Physical activity is a factor associated with maintenance of health body composition. For each influence of exercise below, describe the effect on weight management.

INFLUENCE	EFFECT
-- increases energy expenditure	1
-- promotes lean body mass maintenance	2
-- improves many health conditions	3
-- changes emotional outlook	4
-- differences in responses to exercise	5

Genetic Influences on Body Size and Shape

"...fatness must be considered a multifactorial phenotype, that is the displayed characteristic (phenotype) is the product of numerous genetic and environmental factors."

Use these terms to complete the lists below:

ability to achieve high level of physical conditioning   social influences

basal metabolic rate   taste preferences

economics   thermic effect of food

nutrition   use of ingested fat

Factors that may influence body size and shape (differences in gaining, maintaining, or losing weight) include:

Genetic factors   *Environmental factors*

1._____   1._____

2._____   2._____

3._____   3._____

4._____

5._____

PRACTICE EXAM

1. The following disorder(s) follow the J-shaped curve of risk:
    A. heart disease and strokes
    B. some types of cancers
    C. diabetes
    D. A and B
    E. A, B, and C

2. Following the J-shaped curve means that:
    A. very fat individuals are the only group at risk.
    B. individuals at both extremes of fatness, very thin and very fat are at increased risk.

C. individuals with moderate fatness have the least risk.
D. B and C
E. A, B, and C

3. Restrained eating works against management of body composition because:
A. by dividing or restraining food intake into 3 meals plus 2 snacks, body composition is not managed but manipulated.
B. by restricting food intake below natural appetite levels distribution may occur resulting in bingeing.
C. by restricting food intake weight loss will be too extreme resulting in anorexia-related effects.
D. by applying external measures,a person doesn't develop personal responsibility.

4. Accurate procedures for measuring body fat composition includes all of the following except:
A. underwater weighing (densitometry).
B. bioelectric impedance analysis.
C. anthropometric measurements.
D. none of the above

5. Healthy percentages of body fat composition (essential plus some storage fat) for females is _____ and for males is _____.
A. 20%-25%; 5%-10%; males tend to do more physical work
B. 25%-30%; 15%-20%; gender-specific requirements
C. 15%-20%; 25%-30%; gender-specific requirements
D. 10%-30%; 5%-20%; female needs for childbirth

6. The set-point theory as an aspect of fatness regulation reflects the influences of:
A. physiological factors.
B. environmental factors.
C. psychosocial factors.
D. all of the above

7. Normalizing eating is a key to management of body fat levels. Strategies for normalizing eating include:
A. carefully tracking food intake to limit kcalorie intake.
B. guiding food intake by internal sensations of hunger and satiety.
C. awareness of use of foods for emotional needs.
D. A and B
E. B and C

8. Although exercise is an important component of maintaining management of body fat levels, differences in response to exercise may occur because:

A. ability to exercise vigorously.
B. appetite response to exercise.
C. individual fat distribution patterns.
D. gender.
E. all of the above

NCLEX Questions

1. During adolescence, the greater increase of body fat among girls compared   (PN)
   to boys is because:
   A. the specialized process of that increase the number of cells (hyperplasia)
      occurs during growth spurts.
   B. girls eat more and are less active.
   C. gender differences.
   D. A and B
   E. A and C

2. Individuals who repeatedly diet without success after fuel pressure to try new (SE)
   diets by family, friends, and health professionals. If a client is attempting a new
   diet, a health professional can:
   A. discuss the benefits of exercise (including regular walking).
   B. describe ways to normalize eating.
   C. present the kcaloric values of regularly eaten foods.
   D. A and B
   E. A, B, and C

3. An health promotion approach to maintaining naturally healthy body   (HP)
   composition levels includes:
   A. normalizing eating patterns.
   B. exercising .
   C. following the Food Guide Pyramid.
   D. A and B
   E. A, B, and C

4. Many individuals whose fatness deviates from the usual are comfortable   (PsN)
   with their size and appearance. Others may experience discontent or anxiety
   severe enough to result psychological disorders. These disorders may include:
   A. anorexia nervosa
   B. bulimia nervosa (binge/purge behaviors)
   C. binge-eating disorder (may result in obesity)
   D. A and C
   E. A, B, and C

ANSWERS

Important Terms

1. management
2. body image
3. appetite
4. hunger
5. visceral fat
6. adipocytes
7. hyperplasia
8. hypertrophy
9. densitometry
10. computerized tomography (CT)
11. bioelectric impedance analysis
12. multifactorial-phenotype

Applying Content Knowledge

The body fat levels of Carol and Barbara are affected by their individual genetic makeup that influences their basal metabolic rates and limits their potential to develop lean body mass. Although they perform exercise for the same length of time, the type and intensity of exercise could account for the difference. Both Carol and Barbara are following healthy lifestyle behaviors in relation to body composition and are mostlikely at appropriate levels of body weight and body fat composition.

Quick Review

1. Cultural influence on body image creates a shared concept of attractiveness. Because extensive media coverage the concept of beauty becomes the same regardless of where one lives and acceptable body sizes become limited.
2. Excess body fat tends to accumulate either in hips and thighs or in the stomach area or upper body fat. There re few effects from fat in hips and thighs, but health risks are associated with upper body fat due to the increased rate of turnover. These include higher blood pressure (hypertension), higher level blood lipids (LDLs) and resistance to insulin (increased risk of atherosclerosis, heart disease, stroke, and diabetes).
3. The non-diet approach focuses on long-term changes that results in individuals feeling more comfortable with their bodies regardless of where the weight or body fatness levels change. This recognizes that diets that artificially restrict food intake tend to encourages disinhibition causing bingeing and often weight gain. By developing hunger-directed eating, individuals eat in response to actual physiological hunger rather than emotional or time specified eating.

Body Fatness and Health

1. 1. atherosclerosis
2. heart disease
3. diabetes mellitus

2. 1. menstrual irregularities
2. gallbladder disease
3. some types of arthritis

3. 1. osteoporosis
2. some types of cancer

Body Fat: Essential Versus Healthy Levels

Females -- 12%-14%; 25%-30%
Males   -- 3%- 8%; 20%-22%

Genetic Influences on Body Size and Shape

Genetic factors
1. basal metabolic rate
2. thermic effect of foods
3. use of ingested fat
4. taste preference
5. ability to achieve high level of physical conditioning

Environmental factors
1. nutrition
2. economics
3. social influences

Body Composition and Active Lifestyles

Effect:
1. beneficial effect of daily exercise energy expenditure greater than that of specific kcalories used
2. exercise decreases effect of factors that reduce lean body mass such as aging and dieting; lean body mass uses more energy than body fat
3. reduces the risk of hypertension, coronary artery disease, and diabetes

4. increases awareness and level of comfort with our bodies
5. differences because of factors such as gender and fat distribution patterns; benefits still accrue

Practice Exam

1. E	3. B	5. B	7. E
2. D	4. C	6. A	8. E

NCLEX Questions

1. E	2. D	3. E	4. E

Chapter 11 LIFE SPAN HEALTH PROMOTION:
PREGNANCY, LACTATION, AND INFANCY

"Following conception and continuing until parturition (childbirth), many metabolic, anatomical, hormonal, psychological, and physiological changes take place in the mother."

IMPORTANT TERMS

Match the terms on the left with the correct definitions on the right.

colostrum

fetal alcohol syndrome (FAS)

galactosemia

gestational diabetes mellitus (GDM)

oxytocin

hyperemesis gravidarum

pregnancy-induced hypertension (PIH)

prolactin

teratogen

1._____ an agent that is capable of producing a malformation or a defect in the unborn fetus

2._____ a disorder caused by alcohol consumption during pregnancy that may produce a range of specific anatomical and central nervous systems defects

3._____ severe and unrelenting vomiting in the second trimester or that severely interferes with the mother's life; a serious condition often requiring intravenous replacement of nutrients and fluids

4._____ a sudden rise in arterial blood pressure accompanied by rapid weight gain and marked edema during pregnancy; formerly known as toxemia of pregnancy

5._____ a form of diabetes occurring during pregnancy commonly after 20th week of gestation

6._____ a hormone that initiates uterine contractions of labor and has a role in the ejection of milk in lactation

7._____ a hormone needed for milk synthesis

8._____ an autosomal recessive disorder that results in an inability to metabolize galactose and lactose milk products

9._____ the fluid secreted from the breast during late pregnancy and first few days postpartum

APPLYING CONTENT KNOWLEDGE

"The two outcomes that traditionally have been used to evaluate the influence of maternal nutrition on pregnancy outcome are maternal weight gain and infant birth weight."

Elena Johnson is an 18 year old client at the City WIC program; she is beginning her third trimester of pregnancy. She has attended nutrition education classes taught by the WIC nutritionist. The nutritionist, though, is concerned because Elena has not been gaining suffcient weight to support her pregnancy, but is otherwise healthy. The nutritionist suspects that Elena does not understand the relationship between her dietary intake and the health of her fetus. She asks you, a WIC nurse, to reinforce these concepts when Elena comes in for her monthly checkups. What will you discuss with Elena?

QUICK REVIEW

"The important of nutrition during pregnancy, the benefits of breast-feeding, and the establishment and maintenance of positive eating styles during infancy are crucial to overall health goals."

1.   Briefly describe the major hormonal, metabolic, anatomical, and physiological changes that occur during pregnancy.

2.   Discuss the potential harmful effects on the fetus of alcohol consumption and tobacco use during pregnancy.

3.   Define pregnancy-induced hypertension. List 2 before pregnancy risk factors. List 2 during pregnancy risk factors.

4.   List 4 benefits of breastfeeding.

5.   Breast milk or commercial formula should provide infants with all the essential vitamins and minerals except for possibly iron, vitamin D, fluoride, and vitamin K (for newborns). Explain why these nutrients are exceptions.

6. List 3 potential errors that may occur when preparing formula.

7. Describe the special nutrition needs of a premature infant.

Energy Needs During Pregnancy

"Total energy cost of pregnancy is somewhere between 68,000 kcalories and 80,000 kcalories."

A. Use these terms to complete the following sentence:

BMR   fetal   maternal

The additional energy is needed because during pregnancy maternal

_____ is increased and to provide for the synthesis and support of

_____ and _____ tissues.

B. What is the current recommendation for increased kcaloric intake during each trimester of pregnancy?

Nutrient Needs

"The 1989 Recommended Dietary Allowances suggest increases in all of the nutrients during pregnancy except vitamin A."

Use these terms to complete the chart below:

30	2nd trimester	fetus	red cell volume
56	balanced diet	iron	tissues
180	build	neural tubes	vitamin A
1200	calcium	oxygen	

	RDA/ Pregnancy RDA	Rationale
Protein	1___ g per day/ 60 g per day	Increases to 2_____ and maintain new 3_____ of pregnancy
Vitamins/Minerals	all increase except 4_____	Increase needs but usually provided by 5_____; exceptions are folate, 6_____, and possibly 7_____
Folate	8_____ mcg per day/ 400 mcg per day	Increases aid development of 9_____
Iron	15 mg per day/ 10_____ mg per day	Increase because of maternal 11_____ and iron storage in fetus; supplementation recommended to begin 12_____ ; deficiency impairs 13_____ delivery to fetus
Calcium	800 mg per day/ 14_____ mg per day	Increase meets the needs of growing 15_____

Nutrition-related Concerns:
Diabetes Mellitus, Fetal Alcohol Syndrome, Maternal Phenylketonuria, and AIDS
"Women whose pregnancies are at high risk, such as those complicated by diabetes mellitus, should have early regular nutrition services provided during routine prenatal care; specific education may be needed to sensitize them to their special medical and nutritional needs."

Place the statement numbers next to the correct disorder. Statements may be used more than once.

AIDS/ HIV POSITIVE: FETAL ALCOHOL SYNDROME (FAS) :

DIABETES MELLITUS: GESTATIONAL DIABETES MELLITUS (GDM):

MATERNAL PHENYLALANINE:

1. Symptoms of this disorder cause anatomical defects such as low nasal bridge, short nose, flat midface, and short palpebral fissures.
2. Pregnancy complicates this disorder as the hormones of pregnancy have immunosuppressive effects in vitro.
3. Adjustment of insulin doses may be needed to account for the effects of hormones of pregnancy.
4. If an opportunistic infection develops, increased nutrient needs of kcalories, protein, vitamins and minerals occur.
5. Infants born to women with this disorder are more likely born macrosomic. Even if not macrosomic, these infants require immediate intensive monitoring.
6. If this disorder is untreated during pregnancy, there is an increased risk of spontaneous abortion or serious birth defects such as microcephaly, mental retardation, congenital heart defects, or intrauterine growth retardation.
7. A woman with this disorder needs to continue a low phenylalanine diet throughout a pregnancy to lessen risk of serious birth defects.
8. Pregnant patients with this disorder should be monitored closely for weight gain, nutrient intake, and fetal well-being.
9. The infants of women with this pre-existing disorder are more at risk for major congenital anomaly, particularly if the disorder is not well controlled. These defects may include defects of the cardiac and nervous system such as neural tube defects, kidney, and skeleton abnormalities.
10. Treatment is primarily dietary control combined with moderate exercise that should lead to an appropriate weight gain.
11. Possible teratogenic effects of medications must be reviewed.
12. During pregnancy, adjustments needed to account for increased energy needs. Total kcaloric intake and its distribution will require adjustments.
13. Oral hypoglycemic agents may have teratogenic effects on fetus. Insulin injection is usually required and should be instituted from the beginning of pregnancy or earlier.
14. This condition is the results of alcohol use during pregnancy.
15. The majority of women with this disorder have normal glucose tolerance following delivery, but are at risk for NIDDM.

Energy and Nutrient Needs During Lactation

"A large proportion of the energy stores that are laid down as adipose tissue during pregnancy are mobilized in lactation."

The energy cost of production of breast milk is about 1_____ to 2_____

kcalories per day. Protein needs are higher than during pregnancy; daily

recommendations are 3_____ g/day during the first 6 months and 4_____

g/day the next 6 months. Higher levels of vitamins and minerals are needed but met

through eating well-balanced diets.

Fluid intake is important. 5_____ to 6_____ ml of milk is provided

daily. This fluid must be replaced through 7_____, 8_____, or milk

consumption.

Introduction of Solid Foods

"There are two basic issues when considering the introduction of solid foods to the infant's diet: how to introduce and what to introduce."

1.   At what age may solid foods be added to an infant's diet?

2.   List 2 factors or cues that show that an infant is developmentally ready for introduction to solids.

3.   Why should solids be introduced with a 4 - 5 day interval between new foods?

PRACTICE EXAM
1.   During pregnancy, a woman needs to increase her kcaloric intake during the second and third trimesters of pregnancy by about _____ kcal/day.
    A. 150
    B. 1000
    C. 300
    D. kcalories do not increase

2. During pregnancy, protein needs increase by about _____, requirements also increase especially for the vitamin _____, and the minerals _____ and _____.
   A. 10 - 15 g; folate; iron; calcium
   B. 25 g; vitamin C; iron; calcium
   C. 10 - 15 g; folate; zinc; sodium
   D. 30 g; folate; iron; calcium

3. Nutrition recommendations during pregnancy-induced hypertension include the following:
   A. moderate sodium use of 2,000 mg or less.
   B. well-balanced diet with adequate protein and energy.
   C. limit energy intake to reduce weight gain.
   D. A and B
   E. A, B, and C

4. Strategies for dealing with morning sickness (nausea and vomiting) include:
   A. consume liquids with each meal.
   B. drink fluids between meals.
   C. limit food intake to 3 meals per day with no snacks.
   D. eat more than 3 meals a day by dividing intake into small frequent meals.
   E. B and D

5. Oxytocin is the hormone responsible for:
   A. let-down reflex.
   B. growth of uterus and breast.
   C. relaxation of smooth muscle cells.
   D. prevents premature contractions.

6. Cow's milk is not recommended for infants under 1 year of age because:
   A. it contains less iron.
   B. the fat in cow's milk is harder to digest than fat in breast milk or formula.
   C. it contains more sodium and protein that could lead to dehydration.
   D. all of the above

7. Strategies for preventing baby bottle tooth decay include the following:
   A. bottles given at bedtime or naps should only contain water.
   B. regular cleaning of the gums once teeth erupt.
   C. infants should not be put to bed with bottle of milk, formula, juices or other sweetened liquids.
   D. baby bottle tooth decay is cured by fluoride drops.
   E. A, B, and C

8. The nutrient needs of premature infants include the following **except**:
   A. the same as full-term infants.
   B. increased for a number of nutrients.
   C. possibly met by higher nutrient value in the breast milk of their mothers.
   D. able to be met by specialized infant formulas designed for their special needs.
   E. possibly met by parenteral nutrition or tube feeding depending on their level of suck-swallow reflex.

NCLEX Questions

1. Heartburn during pregnancy may be caused by: (PN)
   A. the action of progesterone affecting sphincter function leading to reflux.
   B. high-fat meals.
   C. growing fetus pressing against the stomach.
   D. wearing clothing that fits tightly around abdomen.
   E. all of the above

2. Client education before and during pregnancy is important; a primary (SE) concern(s) may include:
   A. information about increased nutritional needs.
   B. the potential effects of prescribed medications, over-the-counter drugs, tobacco on the fetus.
   C. the effects of chronic disorders on pregnancy.
   D. A and C
   E. A, B, C

3. Barriers to successful breastfeeding include: (HP)
   A. maternal drug addiction or alcoholism.
   B. maternal common cold or flu or short term antibiotic therapy.
   C. cultural lack of acceptability within which the mother's lives.
   D. A and B
   E. A, B, and C

4. Nonorganic failure to thrive is diagnosed when _____; there may be (PsN) psychosocial causes because of _____, _____, or _____.
   A. organic causes affect growth; congenital heart disease, AIDS, metabolic disorders
   B. no medical reason for poor growth is found; poverty, inadequate maternal-infant bonding, neglect
   C. organic causes affect growth; poverty, congenital heart disease, child abuse
   D. no medical reason for poor growth is found; congenital heart disease, AIDS, poverty

ANSWERS

Important Terms

1. teratogen
2. fetal alcohol syndrome (FAS)
3. hyperemesis gravidarum
4. pregnancy-induced hypertension (PIH)
5. gestational diabetes mellitus (GDM)
6. oxytocin
7. prolactin
8. galactosemia
9. colostrum

Applying Content Knowledge

Because of your age, 18, your body still has special nutrient needs for your own growth. In addition to your needs, your baby or fetus also has special needs to be able to grow and develop fully. This means that the foods you eat should provide enough nutrients for the growth needs of you and your baby. Mothers and their babies are healthiest if the mother gains the recommended amounts of weight throughout pregnancy. This usually means that babies will be born over 5.5 pounds and will start out as healthy as possible. Let's review the Food Guide Pyramid with what you ate yesterday and talk about ways to assure the foods you choose tomorrow will include all the necessary nutrients.

Quick Review

1. Progesterone and estrogen effects are the major hormonal changes. Progesterone develops endometrium and relaxes muscles while estrogen affects the growth of uterus and breast changes. Metabolic changes increase the BMR 15 to 20% to support the increased oxygen needs and tissue growth. Anatomical and physiological changes include the doubling of plasma volume, glomerular filtration rate increases, and relaxation of muscles increase risk of constipation, heartburn, and delay gastric emptying.

2. Alcohol consumption during pregnancy may result in fetal alcohol syndrome or fetal alcohol effects may cause central nervous system and mental defects in addition to cognitive or behavioral dysfunctions and anatomical defects. It is recommended that no alcohol be consumed to prevent any negative alcohol effects on the fetus.
   Tobacco use during pregnancy increases the risk of prematurity, growth retardation, placenta previa, and placenta abruptio. After birth, infants exposed to tobacco in uterine are then more at risk for SIDS, impaired intellectual performance, and decreased attention span.

3. Pregnancy-induced hypertension occurs when a quick increase in arterial blood pressure with rapid weight gain and edema. Two before pregnancy risk factors are family history of hypertension and age extremes such as younger than 20 years old or older than 35 years old. Two during pregnancy risk factors are large fetus and multiple births.

4. Benefits of breastfeeding affect both the infant and the mother. For the infant, two benefits include consumption of immunological proteins and decreased risk of food allergy. Two benefits for the mother include increased facilitation of uterine contractions and easier return to pre-pregnancy weight.

5. Iron may need supplementation because stored iron is used up by 6 months of life. Iron in commercial formulas may not be as absorbable as iron in breast milk and supplementation may be recommended. Vitamin D supplementation may be needed since infants may not receive enough sun exposure to synthesize sufficient amounts. Commercial formula does contain vitamin D but breast milk does not. Fluoride doesn't pass through breast milk. It is only available if water sources contain fluoride and that water is fed to the infant. Vitamin K is a concern only for newborns because there is not yet enough bacteria to synthesize the vitamin. Newborns are usually given a supplement immediately after birth.

6. Three potential errors that may occur when preparing formula include misinterpretation of preparation instructions because of low literacy or non-English speaking; bacterial contamination from the bottle not being sterilized, and adding too much (dilutes nutrient content) or too little water (dangerously increases high renal solute load).

115

7. Special nutrition needs of a premature infant includes problems with suck-swallow reflex requiring parenteral, tube feeding or gavage feeding; increased nutrient requirements for kcalories, protein, calcium, phosphorus, sodium, iron, zinc, vitamin E, and fluids. Special formulas are available that are designed to meet these needs.

Energy Needs During Pregnancy
A. BMR; maternal; fetal
B. 1st trimester no increase; 2nd and 3rd trimesters 300 kcalories

Nutrient Needs
1. 56
2. build
3. tissues
4. vitamin A

5. balanced diet
6. iron
7. calcium
8. 180

9. neural tubes
10. 30
11. red cell volume
12. 2nd trimester

13. oxygen
14. 1200
15. fetus

Nutrition-related Concerns
Aids/HIV: 2, 4, 8, 11
Diabetes mellitus: 3, 4, 5, 8, 9, 12
Fetal alcohol syndrome: 1, 14
Gestational diabetes mellitus: 3, 4, 5, 8, 10, 11, 12, 13, 15
Maternal phenylalanine: 6, 7

Energy and Nutrient Needs During Lactation
1. 500
2. 800

3. 65
4. 62

5. 750
6. 1000

7. water
8. juice (or clear liquids not containing caffeine or alcohol)

Introduction of Solid Foods
1. Solids may be added sometime between 4 to 6 months.

2. Two factors include that 1) the infant be able to sit with some support, and 2) the infant is also able to move jaw, lips and tongue independently.

3. New solids are introduced with a 4 to 5 day interval between each new solid. This allows for isolation of allergic food reactions quickly. The responses may include upper respiratory distress, skin reactions and gastrointestinal distress.

Practice Exam
1. C.
2. A

3. D.
4. E.

5. B
6. A.

7. D.
8. E.

9. A

NCLEX questions
1. E.

2. E.

3. D.

4. B.

Chapter 12 LIFE SPAN HEALTH PROMOTION:
CHILDHOOD, ADOLESCENCE, AND ADULTHOOD

"Once past the very specific nutrition and health necessities of pregnancy and infancy, the rest of the life span categories share more similarities than differences regarding nutrient intake and dietary patterns."

IMPORTANT TERMS

Match the terms on the left with the correct definitions on the right.

anorexia nervosa

binge eating disorder (BED)

bingeing

bulimia nervosa

chronic dieting syndrome

eating disorder

emetic

medical nutrition therapy

senescence

1._____ older adulthood

2._____ a group of behaviors fueled by unresolved emotional conflicts symptomized by altered food consumption

3._____ a lifestyle inhibited or controlled by a constant concern about food intake, body shape and/or weight that affects an individual's physical and mental health status

4._____ a mental disorder characterized by self-imposed starvation; may include binge eating episodes associated with bulimic behaviors

5. _____ a mental disorder characterized as the binge and purge syndrome; includes experiencing repetitive food binges accompanied by purging or compensatory behaviors

6._____ feeling out of control when eating, resulting in consumption of excessive food amounts

7._____ a substance that causes vomiting

8._____ a mental disorder characterized by frequent binge eating behaviors, not accompanied by purging or compensatory behaviors; commonly referred to as compulsive overeating

9._____ the use of specific nutrition strategies to treat an illness, injury, or condition

APPLYING CONTENT KNOWLEDGE

"Children are influenced by and model the behaviors of adults."

Daphne Hawes was upset about the way her young children eat. "Although I have the nanny prepare meals for them, they just don't sit still to eat. They seem to want to just grab foods from the time they get home from school until they go to sleep." When Daphne was asked about her eating style and that of her husband, she responded, "Oh, we both work crazy hours do we don't have time to eat regular meals. We just grab a bowl of cereal or have leftovers from takeout orders." What strategies would you share with Daphne for changing the eating styles of her young children?

QUICK REVIEW

"Each stage of development requires different approaches and is supported in various ways by the larger community."

1. Briefly describe the primary developmental factors of each of the 3 stages of childhood. For each, list 2 factors that influence nutrient requirements.

2. Identify 2 factors that may affect the nutritional status of adolescents. How do these nutritional needs differ from those of children and adults?

3. For the early years, middle years, and older years of adulthood:
    A. discuss an influence that affects nutritional lifestyles of each age category
    B. describe changes in nutrition requirements associated with each age category

4. The eating disorders of anorexia nervosa, bulimia nervosa, and binge eating disorder are described based on categories of psychological and physical characteristics or dimensions. For each eating disorder, list 2 characteristics of the psychological and physical categories.

Community Supports Across the Life Span

"Community supports reveal the commitment of the society regarding health issues."

Match the program or organization with the services it provides.

Child and Adult Care Food Program

Food Stamp Program

Community food banks/ soup kitchens

National School Lunch Program (NSLP)

Corporations

School Breakfast Program

Emergency Food Assistance Program (EMPAP)

State/Local Health Departments

Food and Drug Administration

Summer Food Service Program for Children (SFSP)

Childhood (1-12 years) and Adolescence (13-19 years):

1. _____ provides reduced-price or free meals for children whose household income meet designated Federal requirements
2. _____ provides reduced-price or free breakfasts to needy children (particularly in disadvantaged areas)
3. _____ provides meals to school-age children when schools are not in session in communities where dependent on school meals

Adulthood:

4. _____ provides consumer info (nutrition labeling and control of food quality)
5. _____ provides coupons towards food purchases for individuals with low incomes
6. _____ provides government surplus dairy commodities distributed to low-income households
7. _____ provides bags of food staples to bridge gaps in food availability and hot meals as a food safety net
8. _____ provides community programs on health promotion and wellness
9._____ provide health promotion and wellness centers on site or off site for employees
10._____ provides meals for senior citizens, individuals with specific handicaps, and children up to age 12 who participate in approved licensed day care programs for adults and for children in Headstart, afterschool programs, family day care

Food Asphyxiation

"Asphyxiation from food is possible at any point along the life span, but toddlers and the elderly tend to be more at risk."

1. List two factors that put toddlers at risk for choking:

   a.

   b.

2. Identify 3 foods that may increase the risk of food asphyxiation.

   1.   2.   3.

3. State why the elderly are at risk for asphyxiation.

Lead Poisoning

" Lead poisoning can be an invisible health hazard."

Absorption of lead can be increased by nutritional deficiencies of 1._____,

2._____, and 3._____. Sometimes lead poisoning occurs at the same time as

4._____.

PRACTICE EXAM

1. School age children (7 -12 years) have increased need for:
   A. fat, calcium, iron, and zinc.
   B. protein, potassium, and iodine.
   C. protein, calcium, iron, and zinc.
   D. phosphorus, iodine, and zinc.

2. For adults over 50, the ability to process or synthesize certain nutrients may be reduced. Two nutrients particularly affected are:
   A. vitamin A and C.
   B. vitamin D and B12.
   C. vitamin C and B12.
   D. vitamin E and thiamin.

3. During the oldest years (80s and 90s), malnutrition and undernutrition are a concern. A risk factor(s) may be:
   A. chewing and swallowing problems.
   B. poverty.
   C. impaired activity of taste and smell.
   D. all of the above

4. The _____ phase of medical nutrition therapy for eating disorders provides _____.
   A. testing; a long-term counseling relationship
   B. educational; psychonutritional approach through which the dietitian discusses emotional eating
   C. educational; nutrition information about dietary patterns and nutritional adequacy
   D. experimental; nutrition information about the most healthful strategies for weight loss

NCLEX Questions

1. After age 50, the need for energy _____, while the protein requirement _____.   (PN)
   A. decreases, increases
   B. decreases, remains constant
   C. increases, remains constant
   D. increases, increases

2. Specially trained dietitians implement medical nutrition therapy for eating   (SE)
    disorders. The two phases of this therapy includes:
    A. educational phase.
    B. experimental phase.
    C. testing phase.
    D. A and B
    E. A and C

3. The appropriate age span to begin introducing lower fat versions of   (HP)
    commonly eaten foods is:
    A. 1 - 3 years old.
    B. 7 - 12 years old.
    C. 13 - 19 years old.
    D. during adulthood.

4. Stress may cause physiological reactions that affect nutritional intake or   (PsN)
    status. These include all the following **except**:
    A. excessive adrenaline release.
    B. increase of lean body mass.
    C. loss of appetite.
    D. excessive gastric release.

ANSWERS
Important Terms
1. senescence
2. eating disorder
3. chronic dieting syndrome
4. anorexia nervosa
5. bulimia nervosa
6. bingeing
7. emetic
8. binge eating disorder
9. medical nutritional therapy

Applying Content Knowledge
Children often imitate or model the eating styles of the adults around them. Of particular importance are the habits of parents. Daphne's children seem to be modeling their behavior on that of their parents. If parents use mealtime as a time to enjoy each other's company as well as nourish their bodies, children will view this time as important. If possible Daphne and her husband could try to arrange their schedules so that several nights a week they could all eat dinner together or at least attempt to have one of the parents be available. If that is not possible, perhaps the nanny could join the children for meals and could limit the size and number of snacks so that the children are hungry at mealtimes.

Quick Review
1. Developmental factors of the stages are: Stage I (1-3 years) emergence of autonomy and feeding relationship; Stage II (4-6 years) independent eating styles that are still influenced by adult modeling; and Stage III (7-12 years) preparation for puberty affects growth, moods, and hunger patterns.

Factors that influence nutrient requirements are: Stage I growth and extreme activity increase energy and protein need; Stage II growth and activity levels continue to influence increase energy and protein need; and Stage III protein needs increase depending on maturation (if lean body mass increases) and mineral requirements increase to support bone growth.

2. Two factors that affect nutritional status of adolescents are growth acceleration and emotional/social development stages. The nutritional needs differ at this age category because of gender differences that affect male and female need for protein and energy; these differences are related to puberty that increases levels of lean body mass in males.

The needs of adolescents differ from those of children because adolescent recommendations are categorized by gender. Once past puberty, gender needs vary based on the greater lean body mass of most males. Nutrient adolescent needs differ from adults because teens have higher energy, protein and calcium requirements than adults.

3. An influence for the early adult years is the transition of separating from one's family of origin or from being a full-time student to a full-time employee. For the middle years, an influence is caring for aging parents while career and family demands are still strong. The later years are affected by the transition towards retirement and possible physical or financial limitations.

Changes in nutritional requirements include for the early years, decrease need for minerals due to growth cessation; for the middle years, decrease in energy needs and iron (for women after menopause) but continued need for other nutrients; and for the later years, possible decrease in absorption, synthesis, and processing of nutrients because of the aging process.

4. Psychological characteristics of anorexia nervosa include obsession with shape and body weight and a phobia of obesity; of bulimia nervosa obsession also with body shape and weight and low self-esteem; and for binge eating disorder also low self-esteem and depression. Physical dimension may include for anorexia nervosa amenorrhea and hypotension; for bulimia nervosa weight fluctuation and fatigue; and for binge eating disorder GI tract disturbances and breathing difficulties.

Community Supports Across the Life Span
1. NSLP
2. School Breakfast Program
3. SFSP
4. Food and Drug Administration
5. Food Stamp Program
6. EMFAP
7. community food banks/soup kitchens
8. State/Local Health Departments
9. corporations
10. Child and Adult Care Food Program

Food Asphyxiation
1. a. misjudging size of food pieces
   b. being physically active when eating so swallowing before food is sufficiently chewed

2. 1. hot dogs   2. peanut butter   3. grapes

3. The elderly are at risk because of decreased ability to chew from a loss of teeth or poorly fitting dentures.

Lead Poisoning
1. iron   2. calcium   3. zinc   4. iron deficiency anemia

Practice Exam
1. C.   2. B.   3. D.   4. C

NCLEX Questions
1. B.   2. D   3. A.   4. B.

Chapter 13   NUTRITION IN PATIENT CARE

"During these trying times for patients and staff alike, food becomes very important, both physiologically and psychologically, as it is often one of the few familiar experiences patients encounter in a hospital."

IMPORTANT TERMS

Match the terms on the left with the correct definitions on the right.

branched-chain amino acids (BCAA)

cardiac decompensation

diagnostic related groups (DRGs)

endogenous

exogenous

hypermetabolism

hyporeflexia

hypophosphatemia

refeeding syndrome

somatic proteins

visceral proteins

1. _____ an increase in BMR above expected levels based on age, sex, and body size

2. _____ leucine, isoleucine, and valine

3. _____ classifications used to determine Medicare payments for inpatient care, based on primary and secondary diagnosis, primary and secondary procedures, age, and length of hospitalization

4. _____ originating from within the body or produced internally

5. _____ originating outside the body or produced from external sources

6. _____ proteins other than muscle tissue; for example internal organs and blood

7. _____ skeletal muscle proteins

8. _____ physiological and metabolic complications associated with reintroducing nutrition too rapidly to a person with PEM

9. _____ low serum phosphorus levels

10. _____ impaired cardiac output (reasons not entirely understood)

11. _____ a neurologic condition characterized by weakened reflex reactions

APPLYING CONTENT KNOWLEDGE

"The elderly are more at risk for drug-nutrient reactions because of reduced physiological functional affecting drug utilization."

Danielle Moser, a 75 year old female, is having her yearly physical with her internist. You are talking with her to determine any illnesses or health problems since her last visit; she complains that she hasn't had much of an appetite lately. She also mentions some urinary tract problems for which she went to a urologist for treatment and problems with headaches for which her daughter's doctor gave her some pills; the pills help stop the headaches. You note that neither of these conditions are noted in her chart. When asked about medications for these conditions, she seems confused and can't remember the names of the medications. What should you do?

QUICK REVIEW

"Psychological and physiological aspects of illness, combined with the effects of bed rest and the potential of iatrogenic malnutrition, emphasize the need for nutritional screening or monitoring to identify patients at nutritional risk."

1.   Describe the metabolic response to starvation.

2.   Explain the ebb phase and flow phase of the body's response to severe stress.

3.   Describe 2 immune system components affected by malnutrition.

4.   Identify 2 factors of drugs that affect the use of foods and nutrients by the body.

5.   Identify 2 factors of food and nutrients that influence the absorption or use of drugs.

Refeeding Syndrome

"Refeeding syndromes are associated more with parenteral nutrition than enteral, but discretion and common sense are of key importance in refeeding semistarved and chronically ill patients."

1.   Describe the refeeding syndrome.

2.   List 3 strategies for preventing refeeding syndrome.
      1.

      2.

      3.

Drug-Nutrient Interactions

"Determination of risk for drug-nutrient reactions depends on characteristics of the individual including age, physiological status, multiple drug intake, hepatic and renal function, and typical dietary intake."

For each characteristic below, explain possible effects on drug-nutrient reactions.

CHARACTERISTIC	EFFECTS
Age	
Physiological status	
Multiple drug intake	
Hepatic and renal function	
Typical dietary intake	

PRACTICE EXAM

1. During starvation, the body's metabolic rate _____, becoming _____, while during severe stress, the body's metabolic rate _____, becoming _____.
    A. rises; hypermetabolic; slows; hypometabolic
    B. slows; hypometabolic; rises significantly; hypermetabolic
    C. slows; hypermetabolic; rises significantly; hypometabolic
    D. stays the same; hypometabolic; lowers; hypermetabolic

2. Hypermetabolic stress particularly increases the need for:
    A. protein, vitamins, minerals.
    B. fats, carbohydrate, and fiber.
    C. energy and fluid intake.
    D. A and B
    E. A and C

3. When a malnourished individual experiences acute stress from surgery, _____ may develop causing a very increased risk of infection.
    A. PEM
    B. kwashiorkor
    C. marasmus
    D. hypertension

4. Nutrient absorption may be affected by:
    A. decreased bile acid function.
    B. drugs that increase or decrease motility of GI tract.
    C. development of drug-nutrient compounds that bind nutrients.
    D. all of the above

NCLEX Questions

1. If drug absorption is depressed by the presence of food in the stomach,   (PN) optimum absorption occurs if medication is taken at least _____ hour before or _____ hours after eating or tube feeding.
    A. 1; 2
    B. 2; 2
    C. 1; 3
    D. 3; 3

2. To prevent iatrogenic malnutrition, nursing personnel may do all of the (SE) following except:
   A. contact the registered dietitian to evaluate a patient's nutritional risk.
   B. recognizing that clear or full-liquid diets for more than 24 hours are risk factors.
   C. assuring patients that their appetite will improve soon.
   D. noticing patient's diet orders.

3. Mae Trible is an eighty year-old woman who is on a diuretic for hypertension(HP) and also uses an over-the-counter laxative for constipation. Her appetite is poor, but she is maintaining an appropriate weight for her height. She might be at risk for:
   A. depletion of potassium.
   B. iron overload.
   C. depletion of vitamin C caused by the diuretic.
   D. depletion of phosphorus.

4. Abdul El Marouf is to begin taking monoamine oxidase (MOA) inhibitors. (PsN) He should be educated to avoid consuming foods that contain significant levels of:
   A. sodium such as canned soups, potato chips, frozen dinners, ham, and pickles.
   B. protein such as turkey, dairy products, processed meats, and soybean products.
   C. tyramine such as freshly cooked turkey, salmon, kidney beans, ricotta cheese, and hummus.
   D. tyramine such as salami, pickled herring, beer, fava beans, and aged cheese.

ANSWERS

Important Terms

1. hypermetabolism
2. branched-chain amino acids (BCAA)
3. diagnostic-related groups (DRGs)
4. endogenous
5. exogenous
6. visceral proteins
7. somatic proteins
8. refeeding syndrome
9. hypophosphatemia
10. cardiac decompensation
11. hypoflexia

Applying Content Knowledge

Since the patient, Danielle Moser, is unsure of the medications she is on, the possibility of drug-drug and drug-nutrient interactions is possible as the cause of the anorexia she is experiencing. The internist should be alerted to this possibility and the physicians she saw contacted. With her permission, her daughter could be contacted to determine the name of the physician who prescribed medication the headaches and also the name of the urologist and the diagnosis and treatment of the urinary problem. If possible, this could all be completed while the patient is still in the office. If not, follow-up assessment can be conducted to rule out drug and drug-nutrient interactions as a cause of the anorexia being experienced by the patient.

Quick Review

1. The metabolic response to starvation allows the body to use stored carbohydrate, fat, and protein to meet energy needs. Stored carbohydrate, liver glycogen, is used but is available in limited quantities; it can provide energy for only about 8 to 12 hours. Stored fats, as fatty acids from adipose tissue, are more available providing energy for longer time periods. Because some body cells can only use glucose for energy, and proteins provide glucose more effectively than fats, body sources of protein such as lean body mass, vital organ tissues, or other protein substances such as hormones or blood protein components are used to provide BCAA. As starvation continues additional sources of fats are used to preserve body protein; this may put the body into a state of ketosis. The BMR also significantly slowed to allow energy to be conserved. Damage to body muscles may hasten death as intercostal muscle damage inhibits respiration.

2. The body's response to stress is represented by the two phases of ebb and flow. The ebb phase encompasses the early reaction of the body that begins immediately after the injury. Reactions include decreased oxygen consumption, hypothermia, and lethargy. Cardiovascular functioning and tissue perfusion are primary medical concerns. About 36 to 48 hours after the injury the ebb phase evolves into the flow phase. This phase is noted by increased oxygen consumption, hyperthermia and increased nitrogen excretion. Carbohydrate, protein, and triglycerides are catabolized to meet increased metabolic needs. This phase continues until the injury is healed. Nutrients affected during this hypermetabolic phase include proteins, vitamins, and minerals. Intake of fluid and energy are also critical.

3. Two immune system components affected by malnutrition are GI tract and macrophages. GI tract may allow bacteria to spread from inside the tract to outside the intestinal system. The effects on macrophages may result in more time for phagocytosis kill time and lymphocyte activation thereby reducing the efficiency of the body to prevent infection.

4. Two factors of drugs that affect food and nutrient use are: 1) a drug binding with a nutrient, thereby limiting nutrient absorption; and 2) depletion of minerals if multi medications are used because the interactions of the medications or their individual effects may alter mineral status.

5. Two factors of food and nutrients that influence absorption or use of drugs are if drug absorption is affected by the presence of foods (medications timed with meals or on an empty stomach) and potential side effects of food components interacting with medications for example tyramine interaction with MOA inhibitors.

Refeeding Syndrome

1. Refeeding syndrome consists of complications that may occur when "refeeding" patients with PEM. The conditions tend to occur more often from parenteral nutrition than enteral. As foods and nutrients are increased the excess protein and kcalories can overwhelm the enzymatic and physical adaptation that occurred due to malnutrition. Thyroid and endocrine functions experience rapid changes resulting in increased oxygen consumption, cardiac output, insulin secretion, and energy use.

2. Three ways to prevent refeeding complications include:
    1. Use of a complete nutritional assessment to determine energy needs.
    2. Monitoring weight and fluid balance to assess rate of weight regain and to minimize risk of fluid retention.
    3. Use of refeeding formulas that contain sufficient (but not excess amounts) of all essential nutrients including vitamins and minerals.

Drug - Nutrient Interactions

Age: elderly have reduced physiological functioning that may decrease or alter drug utilization

Physiological status: postoperative trauma or injury may initiate atypical response to medication; effects of weight and metabolic function can affect drug-nutrient interactions requiring more or less medication; careful use of medication during pregnancy reduce risk to fetus

Multiple drug intake: combinations of drugs may alter nutrient levels of body or increase the physiological effect of medications on the body

Hepatic and renal function: if liver and kidney ability to process medications is reduced toxic effects may occur and excretion or retention of nutrients and medications may be atypical

Typical dietary intake: poorly nourished individuals are more at risk for complications because of possible decreased storage of nutrients further reduced by drug-nutrient interactions

Practice Exam

1. B   2. E   3. A   4. D

NCLEX Questions

1. A   2. C   3. A   4. D

Chapter 14   THE CARE PROCESS: NUTRITION INTERVENTION

"All the tremendous advances of medical technology are fundamentally impotent if the recipient is malnourished or is at nutritional risk."

IMPORTANT TERMS

Match the terms on the left with the correct definitions on the right.

anthropometric measurements

comprehensive nutritional assessment

diet manual

nutritional risk

nutritional support

1. _____ the potential to become malnourished

2. _____ a procedure to determine appropriate medical nutrition therapy based on identified needs of the patient

3. _____ determined by simple, noninvasive techniques that measure height, weight, head, arm muscle circumferences, and skinfold thicknesses

4. _____ any nutrition intervention used to minimize patient morbidity, mortality, and complications

5. _____ the reference book that describes the rationale and indications for using a specific diet, lists allowed and restricted foods and sample menus

APPLYING CONTENT KNOWLEDGE

"Patient education can make a difference in patient acceptability of meals."

Bill Kaemmer has had a stroke. Although he is recovering well, he is still experiencing difficulty using eating utensils. Physical therapy is improving his strength and skill, but a modified diet is prescribed to allow for self-feeding. The patient, though, is upset with the foods served and is frustrated by his limitations. His dietary intake has not been adequate. Describe two possible strategies that might improve his situation.

QUICK REVIEW

"For nutrition intervention to be efficacious and successful, a systematic, logical strategy is necessary."

1.   Describe nutritional risk in terms of age, weight, laboratory evaluations, body systems, and feeding modalities.

2.   Identify the responsibilities of the food service delivery systems personnel: director of food and nutrition services department, clinical dietitians, and other staff such as cooks and dietetic technicians.

3.   Compare the nutritional components of a normal diet and a modified diet. Define quantitative and qualitative dietary modifications.

4.   Discuss how the nursing staff can support patients' acceptance of modified diets.

Nutritional Assessment

"Each part of this process is important because there is no one single parameter that directly measures nutritional status, or determines nutritional problems or needs."

The **ABCD** approach of nutritional assessment uses different sources to assess nutritional needs of patients. For each part of this process, fill in the blanks and answer the following questions.

1. A_____ involve measurements of height, _____, and _____.

    A. List 2 reasons for each of these of measurements.

2. B_____ involve measurements of _____.

    A. List 2 _____ parameters and how they are tested.
       1.

       2.

    B. Why should interpretations of these measurements should be cautiously considered?

3. C_____ includes collecting data from several sources.

    Describe 2 sources of data.

       1.

       2.

4. D_____ is collecting information regarding actual and habitual _____.

    A. Discuss a retrospective method for gathering this information.

    B. Discuss a prospective method for gathering this information.

PRACTICE EXAM

1. The nutritional care process uses a 5-step procedure to identify and solve
    nutrition-related problems. These steps include:
    A. assessment and analysis.
    B. testing and training.
    C. planning and implementation.
    D. evaluation.
    E. A, C, and D

2. Anthropometric measurements are useful for:
    A. determining specific health status.
    B. evaluating appropriate nutritional status.
    C. assessing body composition changes or growth over time.
    D. determining the affects of a disease process.

3. The biochemical parameters of _____ and _____ are most important
    because they provide information on _____ and/or _____.
    A. visceral protein status; immune system function; nutritional factors; medical
        condition status
    B. height; clinical assesssment; psychological factors; medical condition status
    C. nutritional factors; medical condition status; visceral protein status; immune
        system function
    D. visceral protein status; clinical assessment; nutritional factors; medical
        condition status

4. Clinical assessment may consider nutritional deficiencies through historical and
    clinical categories. These may include:
    A. avoidance of fruits and vegetables.
    B. abuse of alcohol.
    C. bleeding gums.
    D. poor wound healing.
    E. all of the above

NCLEX Questions

1. Patients are at high risk for nutritional deficiencies when receiving: (PN)
    A. parenteral or tube feeding.
    B. NPO or clear liquids for more than 3 days.
    C. modified diets that affect texture but not variety or quantity.
    D. A and B
    E. A, B, and C

2. To determine if a patient understands the dietary and portion size   (SE)
    recommendations, which of the following would be useful:
    A. 24 hour recall.
    B. ask the patient is he understands the recommendations.
    C. use food models to portray different food portion sizes.
    D. A and C
    E. A, B, and C

3. Acceptance of modified diets is often an important aspect of medical   (HP)
    nutrition therapy. Responsibility for patient acceptance is:
    A. shared by dietitians, nurses, and primary health care providers.
    B. nurses, family members, and patients.
    C. primary health care providers, patients, and dietitians.
    D. dietitians and food service staff.
    E. family members.

4. Willie Johnson, a sixty year old male patient, has been complaining bitterly (PsN)
    about the hospital food. You notice that he has not circled selections for the next
    day's meals from the food service menu. You decide to:
    A. tell his primary care health care provider of his concerns to determine if the
       appropriate modified diet has been selected.
    B. discuss the process for food selection with him to determine if he needs
       assistance in completing the forms.
    C. tell his family of his concerns.
    D. not do anything since his complaints are probably because of anorexia from
       his illness and/or medications.

ANSWERS

Important Terms

1. nutritional risk
2. comprehensive nutritional assessment
3. anthropometric measurements
4. nutritional support
5. diet manual

Applying Content Knowledge

One strategy is to explain to the patient that recovery from the effects of a stroke take time and that he is making progress. He may not realize that the hand exercises of physical therapy will improve his skill with eating utensils. Another strategy is to discuss the purpose of the modified diet that allows him to practice the skills required to use utensils. By providing foods that are easier to maneuver, he will experience success and can then progress to other foods. Contact should also be made with the hospital dietician for further food options that may be more satisfying for the patient.

Quick Review

1. Nutritional risk of age is associated with being older than age 65 (especially over 75 years) or being very young under the age of 5. Weight risk increases with weight loss depending on the cause of the loss. Loss of 5% of body weight in a month or 10% loss in 6 months are risk determinants. During growth, lack of weight gain may be a significant risk factor. Laboratory evaluations of albumin, TLC, and prealbumin levels provide assessment of nutritional status. Body systems account for disorders that affect functioning. This may include treatments that affect dietary intake such as cancer treatments, eating disorders, and diabetes. Feeding modality risk is concerned with transitions from restrictive dietary interventions to regular dietary intake or when modified dietary patterns are continued without regard to possible risk for nutritional deficiencies.

2. The director of food and nutrition services department is responsible for hiring, firing, and supervising staff; ordering and purchasing food and supplies; delivery of food to patients and staff; and quality assurances. The clinical dietitians assess patients' nutritional status, plan appropriate diets and nutrition intervention; and nutrition education for patients. Cooks and dietetic technicians are involved with the actual preparation and portioning of foods.

3. A normal diet is the regular dietary intake recommended for the age category of the patient. It includes a variety of foods and textures. A modified diet is restricted either in nutrients, texture, or quantity to meet therapeutic requirements of the patient as determined by the primary health care provider and/or the clinical dietitian. Quantitative dietary modification refers to the quantity or size of portions served; qualitative dietary modification refer to texture changes to soft, pureed, or liquid forms of foods served.

4. Nursing staff support patients' acceptance by educating patients about their specialized diets and the importance of nutrition as a component of their medical treatment.

Nutrition Assessment

1. anthropometric measurement; weight; body measures
   - A. height - 1. Height is an aspect of evaluating growth and nutritional status of children.
     - 2. Height is used to assess weight and body size.
   - weight- 1. Weight used for screening serious health problems as indicated by changes in weight.
     - 2. Weight levels may indicate over or under nutrition.
   - body measures-1. Skinfold thickness used to estimate body fat stores and distribution.
     - 2. Mid-arm muscles mass circumference indicates skeletal muscle mass. Both reveal aspects of nutritional status.

2. biochemical assessments; body fluids (blood and urine)
   A. biochemical
      1. Visceral protein status tested through levels of serum albumin, total iron binding capacity (TIBC), and prealbumin.
      2. Evaluation of protein intakes tested through 24-hour urea nitrogen (UUN)
   B. Cautiously considered because these tests aren't able to assess short-term response to medical nutrition therapy. Tests reveal most by being repeated over time but this is often not possible. Results should always be considered in addition to anthropometric, clinical data and dietary intake assessment.

3. clinical assessment
   1. medical history
   2. physical examination

4. dietary intake assessment; dietary intake
   A. The 24-hour diet recall involves the patient being interviewed about all foods, supplements (if any), and beverages consumed during the previous 24 hours.
   B. Food records involve the patient writing down all foods, supplements (if any), and beverages as consumed over a specific period of time (usually 1 to 7 days).

Practice Exam
1. E   2. C   3. A   4. E

NCLEX Questions
1. D   2. C   3. A   4. B

Chapter 15 ENTERAL AND PARENTERAL NUTRITION

"Medical nutrition therapy may involve changes in dietary intake to liquefied or pureed foods, tube feeding, or intravenous nourishment."

IMPORTANT TERMS

Write the terms from the list in the correct blanks on the right.

component pureeing

dysphagia

elemental formal

enteral nutrition

osmotic diarrhea

paralytic ileus

parenteral nutrition

percutaneous endoscopic placement

polymeric formula

1._____ decrease in or absence of intestinal peristalsis

2._____ administration of nutrients by a route other than the GI tract, usually intravenously

3._____ anytime the GI tract is used to provide nourishment; often refers to specialized formula feedings

4._____ the inability to swallow normally or freely or to transfer liquid or solid foods from oral cavity to the stomach

5._____each food item is pureed separately then presented in a manner that resembles the original product

6._____ a solution that provides intact nutrients (such as whole proteins and long-chain triglycerides), which require a normally functioning GI tract

7._____ a solution that provides ready-to-absorb basic nutrients, requiring minimal digestion

8._____ placement of feeding tube into stomach via the esophagus and then drawing it through the abdominal skin using a stab incision

9._____ loose bowel movements associated with water retention in the large intestine resulting from an accumulation of nonabsorbable water-soluble solutes

APPLYING CONTENT KNOWLEDGE

"Because of changing health care reimbursement patterns, the demand for home tube feeding has been growing steadily."

Chihae Hsu, a 50 year old female, is to leave the hospital in a few days. She is stabilized on the home feeding regimen and it is time to begin patient education about HEN. Describe the information and skills that you (the nurse) and the dietitian will teach the patient before discharge from the hospital.

QUICK REVIEW

"A clear liquid diet consists of foods that are clear and liquid at room or body temperature, factors that help prevent dehydration and keep colon contents to a minimum."

1. Describe 2 factors of each diet: clear liquid diets; full liquid diets; pureed diets; mechanical soft diets; soft diets; regular or general diets; and diet as tolerated.

2. Identify 3 conditions under which enteral feeding by tube is routine and 3 conditions when it is helpful but not routine.

3. Characterize 3 conditions when parenteral nutrition should be routine and 3 conditions when this form of feeding is beneficial but not routine.

4. Discuss factors associated with successful transitions from parenteral to oral or tube feeding and tube to oral feeding.

Hospital Diet Rationale

"Feeding patients via the gastrointestinal tract is safer, easier to administer, aids in maintaining gastrointestinal tract integrity, and is as much as five times less expensive."

Match the diet with the rationale to the right.

clear liquids diet

diet as tolerated

full liquid diet

mechanical soft diet

pureed diet

regular or general diet

soft diet

1._____ used when diagnostic tests or surgery is scheduled

2._____ prescribed when patients have trouble chewing or swallowing solid foods

3._____ based on patient's ability to chew or swallow, foods processed to smooth consistency

4._____ provides slightly modified food texture with minimal chewing before swallowing

5._____ used during transition from liquid diets to regular or general diets

6._____ used for patients who do not need dietary restrictions or modifications

7._____ permits patients' preferences and situations to be considered

Formulas

"Some formulas are nutritionally complete, some are formulated for specific diseases or conditions, and other (modular) provide specific nutrients to supplement a diet or other formula."

Place the statement under the appropriate heading.

A. can be used by patients with a partially functioning GI tract or with impaired capacity to digest foods or absorb nutrients, pancreatic insufficiency, or bile salt deficiency

B. composed of intact nutrients

C. contain single macro nutrients such as protein, glucose, or lipids and are added to foods or other enteral products

D. may require supplementation with vitamins, minerals, or trace elements

E. meet specialized nutrient demands for specific disease conditions such as diabetes, renal failure or HIV/AIDS.

F. not nutritionally complete

G. predigested formulas composed of partially or fully hydrolyzed nutrients

H. requires a functioning GI tract for digestion and absorption

FORMULAS: Polymeric   Elemental   Modular   Specialty

_____   _____   _____   _____

_____   _____   _____   _____

Feeding Routes

"Patients' medical status and nutritional status often govern the length of the feeding tube (that is, the portion of the GI tract into which the formula is delivered)."

Complete these sentences.

1. When the tube is passed through the nose to the stomach,
   this route is called _____.

2. When the tube is passed from the nose to the duodenum (small intestine),
   this route is called _____.

3. When the tube is passed through the nose to the jejunum (small intestine),
   this route is called _____.

4. When the tube is surgically inserted into the neck and extends to the stomach,
   this route is called _____.

5. When the tube is surgically inserted into the stomach,
   this route is called _____.

6. When the tube is surgically inserted into the small intestine,
   this route is called _____.

PRACTICE EXAM

1. Unsupplemented clear liquid diets are one of the causative factors of hospital malnutrition. A way to prevent this includes:
    A. monitoring of patient by the hospital registered dietitian.
    B. establish hospital policy that diet orders for clear liquid diets are valid for only 24 hours.
    C. when physician's reorder clear liquid diets require justification or selection of more appropriate source of nutrition.
    D. all of the above

2. Methods of administration of enteral feedings include:
    A. continuous infusion.
    B. intermittent infusion.
    C. bolus infusion.
    D. A and B
    E. A, B, and C

3.   Tolerance for enteral tube feeding is optimized by the following criteria **except**:
        A. administering medicine in pill format.
        B. preventing of bacterial contamination.
        C. monitoring patients' tube placement.
        D. temperature of solution.
        E. cleaning tubes regularly according to methods of administration.

NCLEX Questions

1.   Advantages of using enteral feeding include the following except: (PN)
        A. more costly than parenteral nutrition for both the patient and health care institution.
        B. physiologically beneficial in maintaining the integrity and function of the gut.
        C. good for patients able to or willing to eat a general diet.
        D. provide nutrition when the gut is non-functioning.

2.   Criteria considered when a patient is to be an appropriate candidate   (SE)
        for home enteral nutrition (HEN) include:
        A. enteral access is functioning and the patients is tolerating tube feeding regimen.
        B. affordable HEN supplies available.
        C. the nutritional needs of the patient cannot be met orally.
        D. all of the above are criteria.

3.   A normal lifestyle may be possible when patients are able to use home   (HP)
        parenteral nutrition (HPN). Ways to implement HPN to maximize the patient's lifestyle may include:
        A. requiring daily medical care to assure infection free administration.
        B. administering HPN only on selected nights per week supplemented by oral intake.
        C. receiving HPN at night during sleep.
        D. B and C
        E. A, B, and C

4.   A patient on a modified diet is feeling sad because he says misses his   (PsN)
        favorite ethnic foods. He is about to be released from the hospital but will still need to consume a modified diet. As the discharge nurse you arrange for:
        A. the dietitian to visit with cooking and recipe suggestions.
        B. his family to be advised of his concerns.
        C. notify his doctor in case of noncompliance with the modified diet.
        D. A and B
        E. A, B, and C

ANSWERS

Important Terms

1. paralytic ileus
2. parenteral nutrition
3. enteral nutrition
4. dysphagia
5. component pureeing
6. polymeric formula
7. elemental formula
8. percutaneous endoscopic placement
9. osmotic diarrhea

Applying Content Knowledge

The education plan for HEN for Chihae Hsu should include: oral instructions and written guidelines (at an appropriate reading level). The dietitian and nurse need to demonstrate the procedures and then have Chihae conduct the procedures herself. If any family members are going to assist her, they should also participate in the training. Before she leaves the hospital, responsibility for the tube feeding should be clearly assigned to either the patient or significant other (or other family member); this includes the staff assisting in arranging the feeding schedule around the schedules of family members and with consideration of other daily routines. In addition patients may also need sources for obtaining supplies such as formula and equipment; referral to home health agencies is often helpful for provision of supplies and assistance with follow-up visits. The goal is to optimize the transition from hospital enteral feeding to HEN assuring maximum nutritional benefits while maintaining comfort and convenience for the patient. The use of a HEN training checklist is valuable to assure that complete training has been completed.

Quick Review

1. Clear liquid diets:
   1. clear and liquid at room or body temperature
   2. inadequate source of protein, fat, energy, and fiber

   Full liquid diets:
   1. liquid at room temperature
   2. can supply adequate nutrition especially from commercial formulas

   Pureed diets:
   1. food strained/pureed until smooth consistency
   2. can supply adequate nutrition and be modified for special therapeutic needs

   Mechanical soft diets:
   1. food requiring minimal chewing
   2. can supply adequate nutrition and be modified for special therapeutic needs

   Soft diets:
   1. whole foods low in fiber and lightly seasoned
   2. used during transition from liquid to regular/general diet

   Regular or general diets:
   1. no modification or dietary restriction
   2. basis for modified diets and often self-select menus

   Diet as tolerated:
   1. allows for patients' tolerances especially post-operatively
   2. permits patients' preferences and situations to be considered

2. Three conditions under which enteral feeding is routine are 1. major burns; 2. severe dysphagia; and 3. intestinal fistulas. Three conditions under which enteral feeding is helpful but not routine are 1. chemotherapeutic regimens; 2. radiation therapy; and 3. severe renal dysfunction.

3. Three conditions under which parenteral nutrition is routine are 1. bone marrow transplantation; 2. inability to absorb nutrients; and 3. high-dose cancer chemotherapy or radiation. Three conditions under which parenteral nutrition is beneficial but not routine are 1. pancreatitis; 2. major surgery; and 3. hyperemesis gravidarum.

4. Factors associated with successful transition from parenteral to oral or tube feeding include encouraging minimal enteral intake (such as sips of fruits juice) to keep GI physiology normal and maintain gut mucosal. Monitering of actual enteral intake, especially fluids, must be maintained to assure nutrient regimen. Elemental formula use may be required to maintain nutrient status.

   The transition of tube to oral feeding is dependent on assessment of swallowing ability. This is important as transition progresses to full liquids followed by pureed or soft foods. To increase appetite for oral feeding, tube feeding should be stopped an hour before and after meals. Tube feeding should decrease in proportion to increase of oral feeding and completely eliminated after 2/3 nutrition is consumed orally.

Hospital Diet Rationale

1. clear liquid diet
2. full liquid diet
3. pureed diet
4. mechanical soft diet
5. soft diet
6. regular of general diet
7. diet as tolerated

Formulas

Polymeric	Elemental	Modular	Specialty
B	G	F	E
H	A	C	D

Feeding Routes

1. nasogastric
2. nasoduodenal
3. nasojejunal
4. esophagostomy
5. gastrostomy
6. jejunostomy

Practice Exam

1. D
2. E
3. A

NCLEX Questions

1. B
2. D
3. D
4. E

Chapter 16 NUTRITION FOR DISORDERS OF THE GASTROINTESTINAL TRACT

"The ability to chew, swallow, digest, and absorb nutrients, while passing fiber and other substances on for elimination, may be compromised by disorders of the gastrointestinal tract."

IMPORTANT TERMS

Write the terms from the list on the left in the blanks on the right.

chronic ulcerative colitis

colostomy

dumping syndrome

dysphagia

esophagitis

gastroesophageal reflux

hiatal hernia

idiopathic steatorrhea

1. _____ the inability to swallow normally or freely or to transfer liquid or solid foods from the oral cavity to the stomach Crohn's disease

2. _____ return of gastric contents into the esophagus that results in a severe burning sensation under the sternum

3. _____inflammation of the lower esophagus

4. _____ herniation of a portion of the stomach into the chest through the esophageal gap of the diaphragm

5. _____ contents from the stomach empty too rapidly into the duodenum, causing symptoms of profuse sweating, nausea, dizziness, and weakness

6. _____ fat malabsorption as a result of unknown causes

7. _____ an inflammatory process confined to the mucosa of any or all of the large intestine

8. _____ an inflammatory disorder that involves all layers of the intestinal wall and may involve small or large intestine or both

9. _____ surgical creation of an artificial anus on the abdominal wall by incising the colon and bringing it out to the surface

APPLYING CONTENT KNOWLEDGE

"When the musculature of the bowel walls weaken, diverticula often develop, resulting in the condition diverticulosis."

Mark Duffy, a 50 year old man, has just been diagnosed with diverticulitis. He is confused about how he could have developed this disorder because he exercises everyday and doesn't smoke cigarettes or drink alcohol. How would you explain the development of this disorder? Describe appropriate medical nutrition therapy for treatment and for possible prevention of future episodes.

QUICK REVIEW

"Peptic ulcer disease (PUD) is a term for several recurrent chronic disease characterized by the presence of ulcers in the gastric or duodenum mucosal membrane."

1.   Identify 4 warning signs of dysphagia. Describe factors that affect the ability of patients with dysphagia to consume a nutritionally adequate diet.

2.   Characterize the disorder achalasia and briefly describe the appropriate medical nutrition therapy.

3.   What are the combination of factors that may cause peptic ulcer disease (PUD)? Describe treatment goals of medical nutrition therapy.

4.   List 4 symptoms of the dumping syndrome.

Celiac Disease

"Celiac disease or sprue is a chronic disease that damages primarily the mucosa of the small intestine, especially the duodenum and proximal jejunum."

1. Alternative terms for celiac disease may include _____, _____, and _____.

2. Milder forms affect _____, while more severe cases affect _____. Both forms affect _____.

3. The effects are caused by _____ which is found in _____, _____, or _____. Symptoms include _____, _____, and _____.

4. Medical nutrition therapy focuses on _____.

150

GI Disorders

"Disorders of the gastrointestinal tract include those affecting the esophagus, the stomach, small intestine, and large intestine."

Match these disorders with the statements below. A disorder may be used more than once.

dumping syndrome   gastroesophageal reflux
dysphagia   inflammatory bowel disease (IBD)

1. _____ a condition that may occur when part of all of the stomach is removed or pyloric sphincter is removed

2. _____ causes of nutritional depletion include malabsorption, decreased intake of food, increased nutrient use and drug-nutrient interactions

3. _____ management of the disorder requires persistent attention to nutritional maintenance or repletion along with therapies to facilitate healing of the inflamed bowel

4. _____ medically treated by reducing intra-abdominal pressure and gastric acid production

5. _____ major symptoms include diarrhea, intestinal bleeding, abdominal pain, and fever resulting in nutritional depletion

6. _____ patients eat too quickly, stuffing their mouths with food and then choking when trying to swallow

7. _____ remind patients to complete the swallowing sequence before taking their next bite of food

8. _____ therapies may include pharmacotherapy, surgery, and nutritional support

9. _____ ways to avoid condition include elevating head of bed at night, avoiding waist-constricting clothing and not lying down for 2 to 3 hours after a meal

PRACTICE EXAM

1. Way(s) to prevent achalasia include(s):
    A. consumption of high doses of vitamin A and folate
    B. consumption of several large meals a day
    C. no foods or dietary supplements can prevent achalasia
    D. consuming the recommended levels of fiber (20-34 gms)

2. Medical nutrition therapy for peptic ulcer disease provides:
    A. for bland diets especially designed for ulcers
    B. an individualized approach
    C. eliminate foods that increase secretion of stomach acid
    D. A and B
    E. B and C

3. Lactose intolerance may occur as a secondary effect of the following except:
    A. small bowel or gastric surgery
    B. extended use of central parenteral nutrition
    C. acute or chronic diseases affecting the intestine
    D. hiatal hernia

4. Constipation may be caused by organic causes such as _____ and _____ or functional causes such as _____ and _____.
    A. habitual use of laxatives; prolonged bed rest; tumors; spasms of sigmoid colon
    B. lack of fiber and/or fluid; sedentary lifestyle; diverticulitis; intestinal obstruction
    C. diverticulitis; intestinal obstruction; lack of fiber and/or fluid; sedentary lifestyle
    D. diverticulitis; habitual use of enemas; tumors; sedentary lifestyle

NCLEX Questions

1. Adequate daily fiber intake (20-35 gms) keeps the musculature of the   (PN)
    intestinal wall stronger; this reduces the risk of developing:
    A. celiac disease
    B. diverticula
    C. dysphagia
    D. short bowel syndrome

2. Lifestyle changes necessitated by the disorder of _____ involves   (SE)
    using nutrition label information to avoid the _____ found in _____.
    A. celiac disease; gluten; wheat, oats, rye, and barley
    B. Crohn's disease; casein; wheat, rice, corn, and barley
    C. celiac disease; casein; wheat, oats, rye, and barley
    D. achalasia; gluten; wheat, oats, rye, and barley

3. Ways to decrease gastroesophageal reflux include the following except: (HP)
    A. avoid tight-waisted clothing
    B. lying down within 1 hour after meals
    C. elevating the head of the bed
    D. all of the above

4. Patients with dysphagia require: (PsN)
    A. a quiet environment to eliminate distractions
    B. small bites of food
    C. frequent swallowing
    D. A and B
    E. A, B, and C

ANSWERS

Important Terms

1. dysphagia
2. gastroesophageal reflux
3. esophagitis
4. hiatal hernia
5. dumping syndrome
6. idiopathic steatorrhea
7. chronic ulcerative colitis
8. Crohn's disease
9. colostomy

Applying Content Knowledge

Mark Duffy does practice several positive lifestyle behaviors of exercising, not smoking, and not drinking alcohol, but his dietary intake may have put him at risk for diverticulitis. This disorder is tied to a long-term intake of low-fiber foods and it may also be affected by increased intracolonic pressure from straining to have a bowel movement. Both of these may have caused the diverticulitis.

Medical nutrition therapy during the inflamed diverticulitis focuses on allowing the bowel to rest so the infection can heal. Dietary fiber is gradually increased as the inflammation decreases. A high fiber dietary pattern is recommended based on fruits, vegetables, and whole grain breads and cereals; this dietary pattern should decrease the risk of future episodes.

Quick Review

1. Four warning signs of dysphagia are collecting food under the tongue, in the cheeks, or on the hard palate; choking; drooling; and coughing before or after swallowing.

Factors that affect the ability to consume a nutritionally adequate diet include the inability of the swallowing process to be completed; it is hindered further if large amounts of food are taken into the mouth making the process more difficult. The texture of food can be modified depending on the patient's degree of control. Dense and thick foods can be thinned easing the swallowing process.

2. Achalasia is a neurogenic disorder of the lower esophagus characterized by ineffective peristalsis in the lower two thirds of the esophagus, a hypertonic lower esophageal sphincter that doesn't relax in response to swallowing, and esophageal contractions. The appropriate medical nutrition therapy is to serve small, frequent meals of semisolid or liquid foods. Patients may drink fluids with meals to aid movement of food into the stomach. Eating should take place in a relaxed environment.

3. The combination of factors that may cause PUD are hypersecretion of gastric acid, impaired mucosal defense, and predisposing factor of use of nonsteroidal antiinflammatory drugs, *helicobacter pylori*, smoking, genetic predisposition, and stress.

Treatment goals of medical nutrition therapy are individualized for each patient and aimed at reducing intake of foods that increase secretion of stomach acid, make symptom worse, and damage the lining of the esophagus, stomach or duodenum.

4. Four symptoms of the dumping syndrome are epigastric fullness, abdominal cramps, and/or diarrhea that may occur postprandially and vasomotor symptoms of tachycardia, postural hypotension and sweating.

Celiac Disease

1. nontropical sprue, celiac sprue, gluten-sensitive enteropathy
2. microvilli; villi; absorptive ability of the gut
3. gliadin (the protein fraction of gluten); wheat, oats, rye; diarrhea, steatorrhea, flatulence
4. removing gluten

GI Disorders

1. dumping syndrome
2. IBD
3. IBD
4. gastroesophageal reflux
5. IBD
6. dysphagia
7. dysphagia
8. IBD
9. gastroesophageal reflux

Practice Exam

1. C
2. E
3. D
4. C.

NCLEX Questions

1. B
2. A
3. B
4. E

Chapter 17   NUTRITION FOR DISORDERS
OF THE LIVER, GALLBLADDER, AND PANCREAS

"Although they are not part of the digestive tract proper, little digestion, absorption, or metabolism would take place without the liver, gallbladder, and pancreas."

IMPORTANT TERMS

Write the terms from the list on the left in the blanks on the right.

alcoholic cirrhosis

biliary cirrhosis

fatty infiltration

hemochromatosis

hepatic coma

hepatotoxic

jaundice

postnecrotic cirrhosis

Wilson's disease

1. _____ yellow discoloration of the skin, mucous membranes, and sclerae of the eyes caused by greater than normal levels of bilirubin in blood

2. _____ accumulation of triglycerides in the liver

3. _____ neuropsychiatric symptom of extensive liver damage caused by chronic or acute liver disease

4. _____ associated with chronic alcohol abuse, accounts for 50% of all cases , also called Laennec's cirrhosis

5. _____ associated with history of viral hepatitis, improperly treated hepatitis, or hepatic damage from toxic chemicals, accounts for about 20% of all cases

6. _____ associated with obstruction of biliary drainage or biliary disorders, accounts for 15% of all cases

7. _____ a rare, inherited disorder of copper metabolism in which copper accumulates slowly in the liver and is then released and taken up in other parts of the body; as copper accumulates in RBCs, hemolysis, then hemolytic anemia occur

8. _____ a rare disease of iron metabolism characterized by excess iron deposits in the body

9. _____ potentially destructive to liver cells

APPLYING CONTENT KNOWLEDGE

"Each phase of the [liver] transplant procedure dictates specific nutritional requirements."

Michael Singh, a 30 year old male, is on high priority for a liver transplant. He and his family need to be informed about medical nutrition therapy before and after surgery. Explain the medical nutrition therapy guidelines for liver transplant procedures.

QUICK REVIEW

"Medical nutrition therapy is part of the treatment for disorders of the liver, gallbladder, and pancreas; it is also necessary to prevent nutritional deficiencies because of the role of these organs on digestive functioning."

1. Describe medical nutrition therapy for the liver disorders of fatty liver, hepatitis (all types), cirrhosis, and liver transplantation.

2. Explain the differences between cholelithiasis, choledocholithiasis, and cholecystitis. Describe the appropriate medical nutrition therapy for each condition.

3. Define acute and chronic pancreatitis and describe their effects on the body. Discuss the primary goal of medical nutrition therapy and the different types of feeding formats that may be required.

4. Explain why medical nutrition therapy for cystic fibrosis focuses on the provisions of nutrient and kcaloric levels that exceed the RDA.

Liver Disorders

"Nutritional status is influenced by the liver's management of bile production and its role in intermediary metabolism of carbohydrates, protein, lipids, and vitamins."

Complete the table below with the following terms:

chronic autoimmune disease   fatty liver   kcaloric intake

cirrhosis   hemochromatosis   liver failure

esophageal varices   infectious mononucleosis   pale stools

                                                  protein deficiency

Disorder	Possible Cause	Symptoms
1._____	excessive alcohol and/or 2._____, obesity, drug therapy complications, total parenteral nutrition, pregnancy, 3._____, infection, or malignancy	build-up of triglycerides leads to enlarged liver (functioning impaired)
hepatitis (common to all types)	4._____, cirrhosis, toxic chemicals, viral infection	nausea, fever, liver tenderness and enlargement, jaundice, 5._____, anorexia; complications can lead to expanded liver damage and hepatic coma, 6._____ or death
7._____	alcohol, hepatitis, biliary disorders, 8._____, metabolic disorders (Wilson's disease or 9._____), hepatotoxic drugs	portal hypertension, 10._____; ascites, hepatic encephalopathy

Cirrhosis

"Cirrhosis is a chronic degenerative disease in which liver cells are replaced by the buildup of fibrous connective tissue and fat infiltration."

Identify the following complications of the effects of cirrhosis on liver cells:

1. _____ increased blood pressure in the portal circulation caused by compression or occlusion in the portal or hepatic vascular system

2. _____ large and swollen veins at the lower end of the esophagus that are especially vulnerable to ulceration and hemorrhage, usually the result of portal hypertension

3. _____ abnormal intraperitoneal accumulation of fluid containing large amounts of protein and electrolytes usually resulting in abdominal swelling, hemodilution, edema, or a decreased urinary output

4. _____ a type of brain damage caused by liver disease and consequent ammonia intoxication

Gallbladder Disorders

"One of the main constituents of bile is cholesterol, which is also a major constituent of gallstones."

1. List four predisposing conditions for gallstones.
    1.

    2.

    3.

    4.

2. Explain why extreme rapid weight loss is a risk factor for gallstone formation.

PRACTICE EXAM

1. Patients with esophageal varices should be fed low-fiber foods because:
    A. their chewing ability is compromised because of gingivitis and oral thrush.
    B. their digestive enzyme production is limited because of the effect of cirrhosis on the pancreas.
    C. the effect of cirrhosis on the liver reduces the physiological need for fiber.
    D. rough foods could rupture the varices and cause bleeding.

2. Symptoms of intolerance associated with cholecystitis may include:
    A. heartburn, epigastric heaviness.
    B. belching, nausea, chronic upper abdominal pain.
    C. flatulence, regurgitation, indigestion.
    D. all of the above
    E. none of the above

3. Individuals with chronic pancreatitis are often malnourished when diagnosed. The malnutrition is caused by:
    A. overnutrition from the inability to sense satiety.
    B. severe weight loss and malabsorption of fats and protein.
    C. severe weight loss from very low calorie diets.
    D. insufficient consumption of protein and carbohydrate foods.

4. Reevaluation of dietary intakes of individual's with cystic fibrosis is warranted periodically during the life span because:
    A. changes in the disease process may warrant adjustment of nutrient needs.
    B. recommended nutrient/food levels adequately support growth and maintain nutritional status.
    C. weight gain (or maintenance), linear growth, and pancreatic enzymes replacement levels assessed as indicators of dietary sufficiency.
    D. A and C
    E. A, B, and C

NCLEX Questions

1. Although pancreatitis is inflammation of one organ, the pancreas, other   (PN) organs and/or body systems are affected because:
    A. leakage of fluid and plasma from blood vessels supplying pancreas cause damage and edema.
    B. digestion in the small intestine is limited without bicarbonate to neutralize entering gastric contents.
    C. diabetes mellitus can develop if beta cell damage decreases insulin production.
    D. A and C
    E. A, B, and C

159

2. A patient has been diagnosed with a fatty liver condition. The causative agent (SE) needs to be identified and eliminated. In addition to excessive alcohol intake, which of the following factors may also cause faulty fat metabolism?

1. excessive kcalorie intake
2. obesity
3. drug therapy complications
4. TPN
5. pregnancy
6. excessive exercising
7. pregnancy
8. absence of gastric enzymes
9. excessively low protein intake
10. infection or malignancy

A. 1, 2, 3, 4, 5, 6
B. 1, 2, 3, 4, 5, 7, 9, 10
C. 4, 5, 6, 7, 8, 9, 10
D. all 10 of the factors

3. Cystic fibrosis is a life-long disorder. Consequently, health promotion goals (HP) aim to reduce the effect of the disorder and promote wellness. Nutrition strategies include all of the following **except**:
A. RDA levels for kcalories and all nutrients should be exceeded.
B. replacement of pancreatic enzymes to allow for consumption of higher levels of dietary fat.
C. salt restriction is necessary because of excessive retention of sodium.
D. multivitamin supplements (with possible additional use of fat soluble vitamin in water miscible form) are routinely prescribed.

4. In assessing behaviors affecting treatment strategies for disorders of the (PsN) liver and pancreas, which of the following may be the most difficult to assess and to achieve compliance of prescribed behavior modification?
A. alcohol consumption
B. sedentary lifestyle
C. sugar and other simple carbohydrate consumption
D. cigarette smoking

ANSWERS

Important Terms

1. jaundice
2. fatty infiltration
3. hepatic coma
4. alcoholic cirrhosis
5. postnecrotic cirrhosis
6. biliary cirrhosis
7. Wilson's disease
8. hemochromatosis
9. hepatotoxic

Applying Content Review

Medical nutrition therapy recommendations change from before surgery to post transplant procedure. Pretransplant medical nutrition therapy focuses on provision of enough kcalories and protein to reduce protein catabolism and eliminate nutrition deficiencies. After surgery, the immediate posttransplant period of 4 to 8 weeks, individualized medical nutrition therapy is implemented. Complications from surgery and medications such as glucocorticoids necessitate intake of adequate kcalories and protein. If enteral feeding results in inadequate intake, total parenteral nutrition may be required. Regardless of feeding route monitoring of intake is essential. Long-term posttransplant recommendations emphasizes a healthy well-balanced diet. Intake of kcalories, fats, and concentrated carbohydrates may continue to be monitored and possibly restricted if complications of hypertension, hyperlipidemia, diabetes, and excessive weight gain occur.

Quick Review

1. Medical nutrition therapy (MNT) for fatty liver is a well-balanced diet plus elimination of causative factors such as alcohol. MNT for hepatitis is the same for all types and consists of small frequent feedings that are high in kcalories and protein. Carbohydrates can be 40% of the kcaloric intake to promote glycogen synthesis and spare protein. Fluid intake needs to be high and supplements with multivitamins and minerals that contain B complex and vitamin B12, vitamin K, vitamin C, and zinc are usually indicated. Cirrhosis MNT depends on the status of the individual. For example, hepatic encephalopathy may lead to protein restriction to decrease ammonia buildup or other symptoms related to cirrhosis may impair ability to consume and absorb adequate amounts of kcalories and nutrients. Liver transplantation requires different nutritional needs for each phase. Before the transplant, nutrition modification may be followed to decrease further damage from the liver disorder. After transplant, a well-balanced diet with adjustment of nutrient levels as needed is recommended.

2. Cholelithiasis is the presence of stones in the gallbladder. Choledocholithiasis defines the location of the gallstones as being in the common bile duct. When acute inflammation occurs from the stones, it is called cholecystitis and is accompanied by pain, tenderness, and fever.

   In general, medical nutrition therapy focuses on a low-fat diet that is kcalorie controlled; foods that cause gastrointestinal distress are also restricted. During acute episodes, fluids are given through IV and then progresses to solid foods based on patient's tolerance.

3. Pancreatitis is an inflammation of the pancreas that decreases the production of digestive enzymes and bicarbonate and causes malabsorption of fats and proteins. Acute pancreatitis is usually caused by excessive alcohol consumption and gallbladder disease associated with a genetic predisposition to damage. Chronic pancreatitis is caused by chronic alcohol consumption and is noted by chronic pain and exocrine and endocrine insufficiency.

   The goal of medical nutrition therapy is to minimize pancreatic secretions while providing nutritional requirements, particularly adequate energy and nutrients. Replacement of pancreatic enzymes are given and alcohol abstinence is necessary. Different feeding formats may include enteral and parenteral nutrition. Enteral is not used until pain has decreased and GI tract functions without symptoms. Low-fat elemental formulas are used to keep pancreatic stimulation at a minimum. If abdominal pain occurs or pancreatic enzymes increase, enteral feeding is discontinued. Parenteral support is used when enteral is not possible. Peripheral parenteral nutrition is used for NPO of less than 10 days or central parenteral nutrition if NPO for more than 5 to 7 days.

4. The rationale for providing nutrients and kcalories at higher levels than the RDA is that malabsorption of nutrients, pancreatic insufficiency, and frequent pulmonary infections increase nutrient requirements. These conditions deplete or limit the absorption of nutrients and kcalories.

Liver Disorders
1. fatty liver
2. kcaloric intake
3. protein deficiency
4. infectious mononucleosis
5. pale stools
6. liver failure
7. cirrhosis
8. chronic autoimmune disease
9. hemochromatosis
10. esophageal varices

Cirrhosis
1. portal hypertension
2. esophageal varices
3. ascites
4. hepatic encephalopathy

Gallbladder Disorders
1. 1. chronic intake of high fat foods
   2. obesity
3. sedentary lifestyle
4. women on estrogen therapy or using oral contraceptives

2. Very low calorie diets are thought to be so low in fat that the gallbladder doesn't contract enough to empty stored bile leading to the possible formation of gallstones.

Practice Exam
1. D   2. D   3. B   4. A

NCLEX Questions
1. E   2. B   3. C   4. A

Chapter 18   NUTRITION FOR DIABETES MELLITUS

"Diabetes mellitus is a group of conditions characterized by either a relative or complete lack of insulin secretion by the beta cells of the pancreas or by defects of cell insulin receptors, which result in disturbances of carbohydrate, protein and lipid metabolism."

IMPORTANT TERMS

Write the terms from the list on the left in the blanks on the right.

fasting blood glucose

glycosylated hemoglobin (HgbA$_{1c}$)

hyperglycemia

hypoglycemia

polydipsia

polyphagia

polyuria

1. _____ elevated blood glucose levels (> 120 mg/dl)

2. _____ level of glucose circulating in blood serum after an 8-hr fast

3. _____ a substance formed when hemoglobin combines with some of the glucose in the bloodstream

4. _____ excessive urination

5. _____ excessive thirst

6. _____ excessive hunger and eating

7. _____ blood glucose levels that are below normal values

APPLYING CONTENT KNOWLEDGE

"Women with preexisting diabetes who become pregnant are vulnerable to fetal complications, and maternal health can be compromised when complications of diabetes occur."

Mary Jane Goodwin developed IDDM when she was 9 years old. She is now 25 years old and she and her husband are considering having children. Her diabetes, an ever-present aspect of her life, concerns her as she contemplates pregnancy. What strategies should she be aware of when approaching pregnancy with overt diabetes?

QUICK REVIEW

"In addition to the everyday maintenance necessary to control blood sugar levels, diabetes mellitus is associated with disability and premature death because of the disease's effect on structural and functional alterations in many body systems, especially macrovascular and microvascular damage."

1. Describe the microvascular, microvascular, and neuropathy effects of diabetes mellitus on body systems.

2. Explain the relationship of food, exercise, and blood glucose levels for individuals with diabetes mellitus.

3. List 3 goals of medical nutrition therapy.

4. Define the Exchange Lists for Meals Planning.
    Illustrate its use for diabetes mellitus medical nutrition therapy

5. Describe guidelines to use during illness when insulin needs increase and appetite and food intake may decrease.

6. Define gastroparesis.
    Discuss the dietary treatment of gastroparesis.

IDDM versus NIDDM

Place these symptoms and effects of IDDM and NIDDM in the correct columns.

A. blood becomes hypertonic

B. first symptoms are often complication associated with diabetes such as heart attack, stroke, or neuropathic problems

C. insulin resistance or failure of the cells to respond to insulin being produced by the body

D. may be caused by a combination of genetic predisposition, viral infections, and environmental or unknown stimuli

E. polydipsia

F. polyphagia

G. polyuria

H. strong risk factors are family history and obesity

I. significant risk factor of upper body obesity

IDDM   NIDDM

_____   _____

_____   _____

_____   _____

_____   _____

_____   _____

Diabetes Management

"Successful medical nutrition therapy involves the diabetes management team conducting a through assessment, encouraging patient participation in goal setting, selecting an appropriate nutrition intervention, and evaluating the effectiveness of the nutrition care plan."

Assessment

What types of information are collected as part of assessment?

Goal Setting

How is the information from assessment used by the patient for goal setting?

What is the outcome of goal setting?

Nutrition intervention

Describe the types of information disseminated through nutrition intervention.

Evaluation

What is the purpose of evaluation?

How often are additional interventions scheduled for adults and for children?

PRACTICE EXAM

1. Hypoglycemia may be caused by the following **except**:
   A. too little insulin.
   B. too much exercise without additional intake of food.
   C. missing meals.
   D. too much insulin.

2. A difference between the Food Guide Pyramid and the Exchange Lists for Meal Planning is:
   A. that the Food Guide Pyramid was developed by the USDA and the Exchange List by the American Dietetic Association and the American Diabetic Association.
   B. that the Food Guide Pyramid divides groups of foods by their source while the Exchange List categorized groups by each serving containing equal amounts of kcalories, carbohydrates, protein, and fat content.
   C. that the Exchange List divides groups of foods by their source while the Food Guide Pyramid categorized groups by each serving containing equal amounts of kcalories, carbohydrates, protein, and fat content.
   D. A and B
   E. A and C

3. The difference between diabetic ketoacidosis (DKA) and hyperosmolar hyperglycemic nonketotic coma (HHNK) is:
   A. HHNK is caused by an excessive buildup of ketones from use of fats and protein when not enough insulin is available while DKA occurs when some insulin is available but not enough to prevent hyperglycemia.
   B. DKA is caused by an excessive buildup of ketones from use of fats and protein when not enough insulin is available, while HHNK occurs when some insulin is available but not enough to prevent hyperglycemia.
   C. DKA is caused by stress associated with surgery while HHNK occurs from overeating.
   D. none of the above

4. Gestational diabetes develops during _____. Control of gestational diabetes is often achieved by individualized _____. Sometimes _____ may be prescribed to reduce the risk of _____, _____, and perinatal mortality.
   A. pregnancy; dietary plans; insulin; fetal macrosomia; neonatal hyperglycemia
   B. middle age; medication; insulin; hyperglycemia; fetal microsomia
   C. pregnancy; dietary plans; oral hypoglycemic agents; fetal macrosomia; neonatal hyperglycemia
   D. adolescence; dietary plans; oral hypoglycemia agents; maternal macrosomia; hypoglycemia

NCLEX Questions

1. A primary goal of diabetes management, especially for NIDDM, has been (PN) weight management. The latest recommendations include:
   A. new lower weights recognized as most healthful.
   B. reaching and maintaining reasonable weights rather than restrictive weight.
   C. achievement of near normal blood glucose level and desirable blood lipid levels.
   D. B and C
   E. A, B, and C

2. The diabetes management team should include: (SE)
   A. a primary health care provider and a registered nurse.
   B. the individual with diabetes.
   C. registered dietician with experience in diabetes.
   D. A and C
   E. A, B, and C

3. Meal planning for diabetes mellitus is based on: (HP)
   A. a very restricted intake of simple and complex carbohydrates and 50% protein intake.
   B. published diet plans setting levels of kcaloric intake based on ideal weights for height and age.
   C. individualized diet plans that consider food preferences, lifestyle needs, and medications.
   D. predetermined schedule of food exchange units consumed during 3 meals daily.

4. Faulty compliance with medical nutrition therapy for both IDDM and (PsN) NIDDM may be caused by:
   A. lack of knowledge of the disorder.
   B. lack of motivation because of the major lifestyle changes that are required.
   C. lack of motivation because lifestyle changes are lifelong not episodic.
   D. A and C
   E. A, B, and C

ANSWERS

Important Terms

1. hypoglycemia
2. fasting blood glucose
3. glycosylated hemoglobin
4. polyuria
5. polydipsia
6. polyphagia
7. hypoglycemia

Applying Content Knowledge

      Careful planning and devotion are necessary to avoid complications from uncontrolled glycemic levels on the mother and the fetus. Because many fetal abnormalities occur within the first trimester, maintenance of glycemic control must be established before conception. Medical nutrition therapy is primary on a daily basis. Dietary plans should be individualized and take into account the effect of food cravings and nausea. As the pregnancy develops, changing nutrition and insulin needs must be incorporated as placenta hormones and enzymes affect the body's ability to use insulin. A meal pattern that works well is 3 meals plus 3 snacks a day. Frequent home blood glucose monitoring is a positive strategy for tracking normal fasting and postprandial glucose levels. Consideration of these aspects of medical nutrition therapy should assist Mary Jane through a successful and healthy pregnancy.

Quick Review

1. The macrovascular effects include increased risk of coronary artery disease, peripheral vascular disease and cerebrovascular accidents. Microvascular effects focus on nephropathy that affects peripheral circulation resulting in decreased sensation, poor healing to the extent of gangrene development. This nephropathy leads to end stage renal disease for IDDM. Another complication is retinopathy that can result in blindness. Neuropathy complications may cause orthostatic hypotension, tachycardia, gastroparesis, and neurogenic bladder impotence.

2. Food consumption increases blood glucose levels; exercise lowers blood glucose levels. To assure adequate insulin levels to maintain normal ranges of blood glucose levels, insulin intake is adjusted in relation to the amount of food consumed and the extent and regularity of exercise. Food intake guidelines are suggested before and after exercise to maintain blood glucose levels within appropriate levels (not too high and not too low).

3. Three goals are to provide adequate energy for maintaining or attaining reasonable body weight based on age and physiological state; to maintain blood glucose levels within normal ranges by balancing food intake with insulin or oral hypoglycemic agents and activity levels; and to prevent and treat acute complications of insulin-treated diabetes such as hypoglycemia and exercise-related problems and long term complications such as renal disease, hypertension, and coronary artery disease.

4. The Exchange Lists for Meal Planning divides food into groups or exchange in which each group is similar in kcalorie, carbohydrate, protein, and fat content. The groups or lists are carbohydrate, meat and meat substitute group, and fat group.

      Its use for medical nutrition therapy allows for the total amount of food allowed for each day to be divided into specific number of exchanges from each group. From each group the patient can select his or her food preferences while adhering to the total food plan. The meal plan should be periodically reviewed and adjusted every 3 to 6 months.

5. Guidelines to use during short-term illness (up to 3 days) include: monitor blood glucose 4 times a day; test urine for ketones; replace foods if necessary with liquid, semi-liquid, or soft foods consumed in small amount every few hours; and every hour at least 8 oz of fluid, from any source, should be taken. If vomiting, diarrhea, or fever occur, salted foods and liquids should be consumed more frequently to replace lost electrolytes. An individual's primary health care provider should be contacted if no fluid is being retained, ketones are spilling into the urine and/or breathing is rapid or if excessive drowsiness occurs.

6. Gastroparesis occurs to some individuals with diabetes and is more common among individuals with IDDM rather than NIDDM. the effects of diabetes caus vagal autonomic neuropathy. It includes delayed gastric emptying with possible symptoms of heartburn, nausea, vomiting, early satiety, abdominal pain, and loss of weight.

Dietary treatment of gastroparesis includes consumption of six small meals rather than larger meals. Fiber intake may need modifications to reduce constipation or diarrhea and also to prevent bezoar formation that may be common with certain foods such as oranges coconuts, apple, and potato skins.

IDDM versus NIDDM
IDDM: A, D, E, F, G,

NIDDM: B, C, H, I

Diabetes Management
Assessment: Types of information collected include clinical data, dietary history, and nutrition intake.

Goal Setting: The assessment information is used to assist the patient in recognizing behavior changes that the patient is willing and able to make.

The outcome of goal setting is to develop personal and achievable behavior goals related to dietary intake and exercise. The goals are periodically revised.

Nutrition Intervention: The types of information disseminated include an overview and nutrient requirements, diabetes nutrition management, and techniques about menu content, portion size, and carbohydrate intake to insulin levels.

Evaluation: The purpose of evaluation is to determine the effectiveness of the intervention based on clinical data and determination of lifestyle modifications.

Additional interventions for adults are scheduled every 6 to 12 months and for children every 3 to 6 months.

Practice Exam
1. A   2. D   3. B   4. A

NCLEX Questions
1. D   2. E   3. C   4. E

Chapter 19   NUTRITION FOR CARDIOVASCULAR DISEASE

"The term cardiovascular disease encompasses a group of diseases and conditions affecting the heart and blood vessels (1): coronary artery disease (also referred to as coronary heart disease), hypertension, peripheral vascular disease, congestive heart failure, and congenital heart diseases."

IMPORTANT TERMS

Match the terms on the left with the definitions on the right.

angina pectoris

arteriosclerosis

atherosclerosis

congestive heart failure

hyperlipidemic

hypertension

ischemia

primary (or essential) hypertension

secondary hypertension

thrombosis

1. _____ development of lesions (also called fatty streaks) in the intima of arteries

2. _____ thickening, loss of elasticity, and calcification of arterial walls, resulting in decreased blood supply

3. _____ chest pain that often radiates down the left arm and is frequently accompanied by a feeling of suffocation and impending death

4. _____ excess of lipids in the blood

5. _____ thrombus (blood clot) development within a blood vessel of the body

6. _____ decreased blood supply to a body organ or part

7. _____ an average systolic blood pressure $\geq$ 140 mmHg and/or a diastolic pressure $\geq$ 90 mmHg (or both) or is taking antihypertensive medication

8. _____ elevated blood pressure for which the cause is unknown

9. _____ elevated blood pressure for which the cause can be identified

10. _____ circulatory congestion resulting in the heart's inability to maintain adequate blood supply to meet oxygen demands

APPLYING CONTENT KNOWLEDGE

"Several of the risk factors for cardiovascular disease are modifiable or altogether preventable; nonetheless, more than 80% of Americans have at least one major risk factor."

Beatrice Robertson, an African-American female age 51, has primary hypertension for which she take medication; she recently experienced her first stroke. Fortunately, the after effects of the stroke were minimal. Realizing her risk for further cardiovascular disease, she has been exercising with a neighbor by walking for 45 minutes three evenings a week. She finds these walks reduce stress as she often solves work-related problems by discussing them during the walks. Her weight is within a moderate range for her height and she does not smoke cigarettes. Occasionally she will have a glass of wine with dinner. Her blood lipid and cholesterol levels are within desirable range and she has always eaten fresh fruits and vegetables because she grew up on a farm in the South and was used to such a diet. When she first learned she had primary hypertension, she researched which foods contained high amounts of sodium and made a concerted effort to reduce her intake of those foods. Considering Beatrice Robertson's profile, what other modifiable risk factors could she alter?

QUICK REVIEW

" Although CAD has been a public health concern for decades, as health professionals we cannot assume that our newly diagnosed CAD patients, regardless of education or socioeconomic level, are knowledgeable of the disorder and treatment approaches."

1. Explain the use of blood cholesterol levels to assess risk of CAD.

2. Describe the goals of medical nutrition therapy for CAD.
   Discuss the 2-step approach of the National Cholesterol Education Program (NCEP) to achieve these goals.

3. Identify 2 groups that are most at risk for hypertension.

4. Review the medical nutrition therapy for patients who have just experienced a myocardial infarction.

5. List 2 causes of congestive heart failure.
   What may happen to the lungs, liver, bowel, and legs during this condition?
   How may the flow of blood be affected?

6. What is the rationale for restrictions of dietary sodium for patients with congestive heart failure?

Atherosclerosis

"The underlying pathological process responsible for coronary artery disease (CAD) is atherosclerosis."

Identify the correct pathological conditions of atherosclerosis with the symptoms described below.

1._____ when atherosclerosis on the abdominal aorta, iliac arteries, and femoral arteries produces temporary arterial insufficiency upon exertion or ischemic necrosis of the extremities

2._____ thickening, loss of elasticity , and calcification of arterial vessels, from a decrease of blood supply

3._____ thrombosis occurs in a cerebral artery

4._____ if blood flow is partially blocked by a thrombus

5._____ blood flow to the heart is completely blocked

Medical Nutrition Therapy for Hypertension

Lifestyle modifications form the primary approach of medical nutrition therapy for hypertension. Complete the chart below by matching the modification with its rationale.

A. ↑ intake of potassium, calcium, and magnesium C. ↑ physical activity
B. ↓ alcohol intake   D. ↓ sodium intake
                                     E. ↓ weight if overweight

MODIFICATION	RATIONALE
1.	as weight↑, blood pressure ↑; excess abdominal fat ↑ risk
2.	> 2 oz (2 drinks) ↑ hypertension
3.	sedentary lifestyle ↑ risk; regular aerobic exercise recommended
4.	if sodium-sensitive blood pressure may decrease
5.	↑ intake of potassium, calcium, and magnesium ↓ risk of hypertension

PRACTICE EXAM

1. Total blood cholesterol is frequently used to assess coronary artery disease risk. Cholesterol levels are affected by:
    A. physical activity.
    B. genetic factors.
    C. saturated fat and cholesterol content of the diet.
    D. obesity.
    E. all of the above

2. In about _____ of hypertension is _____ because the cause is unknown.
    A. 50%; primary or essential
    B. 50%; secondary or essential
    C. 95%; primary or essential
    D. 95%; secondary or essential

3. _____ hypertension may be caused by _____ disorders, Cushing's syndrome and primary aldosteronism.
    A. secondary; renal
    B. secondary; adrenal
    C. primary; renal
    D. primary; pancreas

NCLEX Questions

1. Congestive heart failure may substantially increase energy needs over basal (PN) needs because:
    A. inability to digest foods well because of reduction of digestive functions.
    B. liver functions requires additional energy.
    C. increased cardiac and pulmonary energy needs.
    D. all of the above

2. Patients on sodium restricted diets need to be aware of the symptoms of (SE) hyponatremia. These may include:
    A. muscle cramps ad weakness.
    B. hypotension and oliguria.
    C. tiredness and disorientation.
    D. all of the above

3. The risk factors of cardiovascular disease are divided into 3 groups of   (HP)
    controllable, noncontrollable, and predisposing conditions. Predisposing
    conditions may include:
    A. diabetes mellitus, age, tobacco use, and hypertension.
    B. diabetes mellitus, hypertension, and hypercholesterolemia.
    C. tobacco use, hypertension, and gender.
    D. tobacco use, diabetes mellitus, physical activity.

4. The elderly may need additional support on antihypertensive and reduced-   (PsN)
    sodium diets because:
    A. dietary modifications may be understood as restricting total food intake.
    B. risk is higher for dehydration and orthostatic hypertension.
    C. specific taste preferences should be considered in formulating food patterns to
        support compliance.
    D. A, B, and C
    E. A and C

ANSWERS

Important Terms

1. atherosclerosis
2. arteriosclerosis
3. angina pectoris
4. hyperlipidemic
5. thrombosis
6. ischemia
7. hypertension
8. primary (or essential) hypertension
9. secondary hypertension
10. congestive heart failure

Applying Content Knowledge

Beatrice Robertson is already addressing the controllable risk factors of tobacco use and physical inactivity. The predisposing condition of hypertension is being treated by her primary care provider and other potential predisposing conditions of obesity, diabetes mellitus, and hypercholesterolemia are either being addressed or are not an issue for Beatrice.

Quick Review

1. The risk of coronary artery disease increases as the blood cholesterol levels rise. Low density lipoproteins present the most accurate level of cholesterol concentration traveling in the blood because they contain 60%-70% of the total serum cholesterol. Nonetheless, total blood cholesterol can still provide an assessment of risk particularly if levels are over 200 mg/dl.

2. The goals of medical nutrition therapy for CAD include reducing total fat, saturated fat, and cholesterol dietary intake to reduce total cholesterol, LDL-cholesterol, and triglyceride levels.

The 2-step approach of the National Cholesterol Education Program is to implement the goals of medical nutrition therapy. Step 1 provides for total kcaloric intake to be 30% or less from total fats, 8% to 10% total kcalories from saturated fats; with 10 or less from polyunsaturated fats; and 15% or less from monounsaturated fats. Carbohydrate intake is to be 55% or less of total kcaloric intake and protein at about 15% of total kcalories. Cholesterol intake is to be less than 300 mg/day. Differences in Step 2 are that the level of saturated fats is reduced to less than 7% of total kcalories and intake of cholesterol is lowered to 200 mg/day or less. Otherwise other levels are the same for both including a recommendation for total kcaloric intake to be achieve and maintain desirable weight.

3. Two groups that are at risk for hypertension are people with lower educational and income levels and non-Anglo-Americans including African-American, Puerto Ricans, Cuban-Americans, and Mexican Americans.

4. Patients after a myocardial infarction receive a liquid diet for the first 24 hours. Foods are gradually offered. Small, frequent meals put less stress on the heart by not increasing splanchnic blood flow. To avoid myocardial stimulation caffeinated beverages are avoided as are food and beverages that are very hot or very cold. Other aspects of dietary intake are controlled based on the individual needs of the patients; these include sodium, cholesterol, fat, and kcalories. Consumption of foods containing omega-3 fatty acids may help to reduce the risk of blood clots. Good sources of omega-3 fatty acids are tuna, salmon, halibut, sardines, and lake trout.

5. Two causes of congestive heart failure are CAD and lung disease.
   The lungs, liver, bowel, and legs may develop congestion and edema.
   Blood flow may decrease to the kidneys leading to retention of sodium and fluid.

6. Sodium is restricted for patients with congestive heart failure because this restriction reduces the workload of the heart. Restricting sodium lessens the levels of extracellular fluids, thereby easing the efforts required of the heart.

Atherosclerosis
1. peripheral vascular disease   3. cerebrovascular accident or stroke   5. myocardial infarction
2. arteriosclerosis   4. angina pectoris

Medical Nutrition Therapy for Hypertension
1. E   2. B   3. C   4. D   5. A

Practice Exam
1. E   2. C   3. A

NCLEX Questions
1. C   2. D   3. B   4. D

Chapter 20   NUTRITION FOR DISEASES OF THE KIDNEYS

"The chief, life-preserving function of the kidneys is to maintain chemical homeostasis in the body."

IMPORTANT TERMS

Write the terms from the list in the correct blanks on the right.

anuria

azotemia

hemodialysis

heparinized

nephrosclerosis

oliguria

peritoneal dialysis

recombinant EPO

uremia

uremic toxicity

1._____ < 400 ml urine excretion/24 hr

2. _____ < 250 ml urine excretion/24 hr

3. _____ retention of excessive amounts of nitrogenous compounds in the blood caused by the kidney's failure to remove urea from the blood

4. _____ necrosis of the renal arterioles, associated with hypertension

5. _____ excessive amounts of urea and other nitrogenous waste products in the blood

6._____ a procedure to remove impurities or wastes from the blood in treating renal insufficiency by shunting the blood from the body through a machine for diffusion and ultrafiltration and then returned to the patient's circulation

7. _____ a dialysis procedure performed to correct an imbalance of fluid or electrolytes in the blood or other wastes by using the peritoneum as the diffusible membrane

8. _____ buildup of toxic waste products (urea and other nitrogenous waste) in the blood

9. _____ use of an antithrombin factor to prevent intravascular clotting

10. _____ recombinant human erythropoietin; drug used to treat anemia by replacing erythropoietin for patients with CRF who do not produce this hormone in adequate amounts

179

APPLYING CONTENT KNOWLEDGE

"Dietary habits can increase the risk of stone formation in susceptible persons."

Joe Romano, a 40 year old male, has just been diagnosed with kidney stones. His mother and aunt also had kidney stones. When questioned about his dietary intake, Joe seems surprised, asking what that has to do with kidney stones. A review of his diet and supplement intake reveals that Joe often doesn't drink many fluids during the day because his job limits his access to beverages. His dietary intake includes a high percentage of protein because he feels that meat and chicken keep him strong. He consumes few foods that contain calcium and tends to eat snack and processed foods that are salty. In addition to his beliefs about protein, he believes that vitamin C keeps him from developing colds so every day he ingests 1500 mg of vitamin C. What general dietary advice should be discussed with Joe Romano to reduce his risk of developing future stones?

QUICK REVIEW

"Various inflammatory, obstructive, and degenerative diseases affect the kidneys in different ways. These disorders interfere with the normal functioning of the nephrons to regulate products of body metabolism."

1. Discuss the goals of medical nutrition therapy for nephrotic syndrome.

2. List 3 common causes of acute renal failure (ARF).
    Identify how nutritional needs are determined.

3. List 3 potential causes of chronic renal failure (CRF).
    When CRF progresses to end stage renal disease (ESRD), identify the treatment modalities used to reduce uremia.

4. Describe the purpose of the National Renal Diet.

5. Explain the difference between hemodialysis and peritoneal dialysis.

6. Review the objectives of medical nutrition therapy for peritoneal dialysis.
    Compare nutrient needs with those required for hemodialysis.

7. Discuss the immediate and long-term posttransplant nutrient needs of patients receiving renal transplants.

Nephrotic Syndrome

"Nephrotic syndrome is a term used to describe a complex of symptoms that can occur as a result of damage to the capillary walls of the glomerulus."

Match the terms below with the description of symptoms of nephrotic syndrome.

A. glomerulonephritis   C. hypoalbuminemia   E. proteinuria
B. hyperlipidemia   D. lupus erythematosus

1. _____ >3-3.5 gm protein lost in urine daily

2. _____ decreased serum levels of albumin

3. _____ the name of a group of diseases that damage the renal glomeruli

4. _____ a chronic inflammatory disease of unknown cause that affects many body systems

5. _____ elevated serum lipid levels

Acute Renal Failure

"Although a few patients do not experience any reduction in urine output, two thirds experience the following three stages: oliguric, diuretic, and recovery."

Identify the three stages and their duration. Place in the appropriate column.

diuretic   7 to 14 days
oliguric   7 to 21 days
recovery   about 3 to 12 months

STAGE	DURATION	SYMPTOMS
1.	2.	- azotemia, acidosis, high serum potassium, high serum phosphorus, hypertension, anorexia, edema, and risk of water intoxication
3.	4.	- urine output gradually ↑
5.	6.	- kidney function gradually improves; may be some residual permanent damage

Hemodialysis: Nutrient Needs

"During hemodialysis, blood is removed by way of a special vascular access or shunt (usually in the nondominant forearm), heparinized, cleansed of excess fluid and waste products through a semipermeable membrane, and then returned to the patient's circulation."

Complete the sentences below with these terms. (Terms may be used more than once.)

calcium   fat-soluble   iron   phosphorus   water-soluble   vitamin D

Patients who are receiving hemodialysis are routinely restricted in the 1._____ content of their diets. High levels of serum 2._____ contribute to secondary hyperparathyroidism and raise the calcium- 3._____ product in the plasma.

4._____ often needs to be supplemented. Impaired 5._____ absorption is caused by the lack of the active form of 6._____ (calcitriol) and prescribed diets are usually low in 7._____ because dairy products are restricted because of the high 8._____ content. Still, serum levels should be monitored for hypercalcemia.

Kidneys, during renal failure, lose the ability perform an endocrine function of producing calcitriol, the active form of 9._____. It is only the active form that provides protection from bone disease; it is supplemented in an oral form or IV form during hemodialysis.

Another endocrine function affected by CRF is decreased production of the hormone erythropoietin that stimulates bone marrow to produce red blood cells. 10._____ supplementation is often required to provide a sufficient supply for erythropoiesis production. Recombinant erythropoietin can be provided during dialysis or subcutaneously just after dialysis treatment.

Deficiencies of 11._____ vitamins are also possible, particularly vitamin B6 and folic acid; these deficiencies may occur because of a low intake or loss during dialysis. Supplementation of 12._____ vitamins is usually not necessary.

Renal Calculi

"Most calculi are composed of calcium, oxalate, or phosphorus, with a small proportion formed from cystine or uric acid."

A. Identify the four factors that lead to formation of kidney stones:

    1.   3.

    2.   4.

B. 1. To reduce the risk of calcium stones, should the calcium or oxalate content of the diet be controlled? Why?

    2. What foods and supplements should be restricted?

PRACTICE EXAM

1. Goals of medical nutrition therapy for nephrotic syndrome include all of the following **except**:
   A. reduce edema and decrease urinary albumin losses.
   B. prevent protein malnutrition and muscle breakdown.
   C. control hypotension.
   D. provide adequate energy.

2. Determinants of nutritional needs during acute renal failure depends on the cause of ARF. Patients will be _____ if the cause was burns, _____, infection, or _____.
   A. hypermetabolic; trauma; septicemia
   B. hypermetabolic; genetic; septicemia
   C. hypometabolic; trauma; septicemia
   D. hypometabolic; trauma; dialysis

3. Reducing intake of _____ and _____ to minimum requirement can slow the progress of chronic renal failure.
   A. potassium; carbohydrates
   B. potassium; lipids
   C. protein; phosphorus
   D. protein; zinc

4. During renal failure the kidneys lose their endocrine function of producing _____; this may affect bone health.
   A. insulin
   B. calcitriol
   C. thyroxine
   D. glucagon

5. During peritoneal dialysis, restriction of _____ is necessary to prevent _____.
   A. water; osteoporosis
   B. sodium; osteomalacia
   C. phosphorus; rickets
   D. phosphorus; osteodystrophy

NCLEX Questions

1. Symptoms of uremic toxicity due to chronic renal failure include all of the (PN) following **except**:
   A. nausea.
   B. metallic taste in the mouth.
   C. anorexia.
   D. increased appetite.
   E. lethargy.

2. Medical nutrition therapy for nephrotic syndrome usually requires restricting (SE) sodium to help control hypertension and edema. Patients may not be aware of hidden sources of sodium such as:
   A. toothpaste.
   B. mouthwash.
   C. water supply.
   D. medications.
   E. all of the above

3. Preventive strategies for decreasing risk of kidney stones include: (HP)
   A. increase intake of potassium by eating more fruits and vegetables.
   B. limit foods high in oxalates.
   C. limit intake of water and other fluids.
   D. A and B
   E. A, B, and C

4. Adherence to specialized dietary recommendations are crucial to the success(PsN) of medical nutrition therapy for diseases of the kidneys.
   The National Renal Diet supports compliance by:
   A. allowing meal plan designs that meets the specific needs of each patient.
   B. providing a framework for patient education.
   C. recommending vegetarian dietary patterns.
   D. A and B
   E. A, B, and C

ANSWERS

Important Terms

1. oliguria	4. nephrosclerosis	7. peritoneal dialysis
2. anuria	5. uremia	8. uremic toxicity
3. azotemia	6. hemodialysis	9. heparinized
		10. recombinant EPO

Applying Content Knowledge

Since Joe Romano is clearly susceptible to kidney stones, he can implement some dietary changes to reduce his future risk. He needs some strategies to increase his liquid intake during the day. Perhaps he can schedule some breaks for drinks or can bring some portable sources of fluid with him to his work environment. Reducing his animal protein intake will also reduce risk by decreasing urinary uric acid. By increasing his calcium food intake, the amount of oxalate absorbed is reduced, so less oxalate is excreted in the urinary tract. Risk for kidney stones will also be decreased by consuming less sodium so substituting salty snacks with other foods such as those higher in calcium is important. Finally, he should reduce his intake of vitamin C supplements slowly to prevent a rebound effect and to decrease its effect on urinary oxalate excretion.

Quick Review

1. The goals of medical nutrition therapy are to decrease edema, reduce urinary albumin losses, control hypertension, prevent protein malnutrition and muscle wasting, while supplying adequate energy, and slowing the progression of the disease. To achieve these goals, patients need to consume sufficient amounts of protein of .8 to 1.0 g/kg/day and of kcalories at ≥35 kcal/kg/day. Most of the kcalories should be from carbohydrates at 50% to 60% of total kcal and monounsaturated and polyunsaturated fats are suggested because of risk of hyperlipidemia. Dietary sodium can be limited to reduce hypertension and edema; education about sodium levels of foods, medications, and even water supply may be necessary.

2. Three common causes of ARF are septicemia, hemorrhage and streptococcal infection.
   Nutritional needs are determined by whether or not dialysis is used and what is the underlying cause of ARF. If caused by trauma, burns septicemia, or infection, patients may be hypermetabolic, which will affect nutritional needs. Also, needs fluctuate, depending on the stage the patient is in.

3. Three potential causes of CRF are nephrosclerosis, obstructive diseases, and diabetes mellitus.
   Treatment modalities used to reduce uremia are conservative management, hemodialysis, peritoneal dialysis, and renal transplantation.

4. The National Renal Diet was developed by the Renal Dietitians' Practice Group and the National Kidney Foundation Council on Renal Nutrition to provide a renal diet that could be used anywhere in the United States. Ethnic variability is not included but can be added as the dietary recommendations are intended to be a starting point for individualizing diet plans. The aim is to increase patient compliance by providing meal plans to meet specific needs.

5. The the difference between hemodialysis and peritoneal dialysis is that hemodialysis is a process through which blood is removed through a special vascular shunt or access, heparinized, cleaned through a semipermeable membrane of excess fluid and wastes, and then returned to the patient's circulation. With peritoneal dialysis the peritoneal membrane functions as the filter. Waste products and excess fluid are discarded through a surgially placed catheter.

6. The objectives of medical nutrition therapy for peritoneal dialysis (PD) are to maintain nutritional status while returning lost albumin (from the dialysate), mimimisze complications of fluid and metabolic imbalances, and reduce symptoms of uremic toxicity .

Differences of nutritional needs are that with hemodialysis, patients tend to have **higher energy needs** because patients treated with PD receive additional kcalories from the PD dialysate. As with hemodialysis, patients undergoing PD are at risk for water-soluble vitamins and mineral deficiencies so that supplementation is recommended.

7. The immediate nutrient needs are that kcalorie needs are high because of stress from surgery and breakdown of body tissues. Long-term posttransplant needs reduce energy needs at about 6 to 8 weeks after the transplant. The aim is to maintain desirable body weight. Dietary protein does not need to be restricted and may need to be increased. Effects of medications may necessitate restriction of simple carbohydrates if glucose intolerance develops and fats may need limitations if hypercholesterolemia and/or hypertriglyceridemia develop. Other restrictions may develop based on reactions to medications used posttransplantation.

Nephrotic Syndrome
1. E   2. C   3. A   4. D   5. B

Acute Renal Failure
1. oliguric   3. diuretic   5. recovery
2. 7 to 21 days   4. 7 to 14 days   6. about 3 to 12 months

Hemodialysis: Nutrient Needs
1. phosphorus   4. calcium   7. calcium   10. iron
2. phosphorus   5. calcium   8. phosphorus   11. water-soluble
3. phosphorus   6. vitamin D   9. vitamin D   12. fat-soluble

Renal Calculi
A. 1. low urine volume   3. excessive urinary excretion of calcium, oxalate, uric acid, or a combination
   2. high urine pH   4. decreased levels of substances in urine that usually inhibit stone formation

B. 1. The oxalate content should be reduced. Calcium stone formation has been linked with higher oxalate in the urinary tract. If the calcium content of diet is kept high, the calcium can bind oxalate so that less is absorbed.
   2. Specific foods that should be avoided because they increase urinary oxalate excretion are spinach, rhubarb, beets, nuts, chocolate, tea, wheat bran, and strawberries. Protein and sodium intake should be moderate and vitamin C supplements should be avoided (may increase urinary oxalate excretion).

Practice Exam
1. C   2. A   3. C   4. B   5. D

NCLEX Questions
1. D   2. E   3. D   4. D

Chapter 21 NUTRITION IN CANCER, AIDS,
AND OTHER SPECIAL PROBLEMS

"...the nutritional status of patients with cancer, acquired immune deficiency syndrome, and/or pulmonary disease is challenged by manifestations not only of the disease, but by the ramifications of treatment as well."

IMPORTANT TERMS
Write the terms from the list in the correct blanks on the right.

antineoplastic therapy

benign neoplasm

cancer

cancer cachexia

fractionation

malignant neoplasm

neutropenia

retrovirus

1. _____ uncontrolled growth of cells that tend to invade surrounding tissue and metastasize to distant body sites

2. _____ a tumor of limited growth, defined shape; does not spread to surrounding tissue or other body organs

3. _____ a tumor that grows in an uncontrolled manner invading surrounding tissue, metastasizes and may cause death if untreated

4. _____ substance, procedure, or measure that prevents the proliferation of malignant cells; usually chemotherapy, radiation therapy, surgery, biologic response modifiers, bone marrow transplantation

5. _____ a syndrome due to a malignant tumor characterized by anorexia, alterations in taste sensation, weight loss, anemia, weakness, and emaciation which results in decline of physical and mental functions

6. _____ administration of radiation in smaller doses over time rather than in one large dose

7. _____ abnormally low levels of circulating white blood cells that remove bacteria

8. _____ an RNA virus that becomes integrated into the DNA of a host cell during replication

189

APPLYING CONTENT KNOWLEDGE

As part of nutrition intervention for cancer patients: *"Assess meal patterns and snacks. Previous dietary restrictions (for example , cholesterol, fat, and total kcalories) may need to be liberalized. Patients may hesitate to eat between meals or eat high-kcalorie foods. Inform patients and significant others that these dietary restrictions are no longer necessary."*

Meryl Crystal, a 45 year-old female, is recovering from surgery for breast cancer. Chemotherapy has been difficult resulting in nausea and vomiting; the patient had been losing weight. But during this visit, you note that her weight is stable. During questioning about her diet history, she reveals that she saw a naturopathic doctor. He developed a dietary plan to reduce the symptoms related to chemotherapy. This plan included instructions that she avoid certain foods because of their acidic content and that she ease up on her personal restrictions on the number of kcalories and amount of fat she consumes. Meryl also explains that she continued her usual strict weight loss maintenance regimen once she left the hospital but is now following the recommendations of the naturopathic doctor. You look over the diet and note that just a few fruits and vegetables are eliminated and that some varieties of beef and fish are limited in serving size. What are 2 possible concerns to discuss with Meryl and what recommendations could be provided?

QUICK REVIEW

"Most of the medical nutrition therapy prescribed focuses on reducing these effects and supporting patients through the potentially debilitating side-effects of treatment."

1.   Describe the diet/cancer connection.

2.   Identify 4 nutritional interventions for patients with cancer.

3.   List 4 warning signs of factors that may negatively affect nutritional status of patients with HIV/AIDS.

4.   Describe the medical nutrition therapy prescribed for pulmonary disease disorders.

Nutritional Effects of Cancer Therapy

"Local or systemic effects of the cancer combined with antineoplastic therapy place the patient with cancer at increased risk of developing malnutrition or the wasting syndrome of cancer cachexia."

Complete the chart using these terms:

bacterial and fungal infections   chemotherapy   learned food aversions

bone marrow transplantation   dumping syndrome   radiation therapy

                                          surgery

Cancer Treatment	Sites Primarily Affected	Symptoms Altering Nutritional Status
1. _____	all cells; most affected bone marrow and cells of GI tract	anorexia; nausea; vomiting; mucositis; stomatitis; organ injury; 2. _____
3. _____	region or area of body radiated; primary sites of head and neck, abdomen and pelvis (GI tract), and central nervous system	anorexia; nausea; vomiting; stomatitis; esophageal mucositis; loss of taste sensation; dry mouth; malabsorption; diarrhea; steatorrhea, ulceration; bowel damage or obstruction
4. _____	GI tract (removal of tumors)	malabsorption; diarrhea; steatorrhea; 5. _____ hypoglycemia
6. _____	immune system; all cells possibly affected by pre-transplant treatment with chemotherapy; possible damage to skin, GI tract, and liver if graft versus host disease develops	potential of 7. _____ (from fruits and vegetables); stomatitis; taste changes; xerostomia; anorexia

AIDS and Malnutrition

"Occurring in 80% or more of people with HIV/AIDS, the development of malnutrition is multifactorial, ranging from decreased nutrient (food) intake, malabsorption, and altered metabolism."

For each category below, identify 2 symptoms or determinants that affect nutritional status of individual s with HIV/AIDS:

Physical Symptoms	*Psychosocial Determinants*	*Economic Considerations*
1._____	3._____	5._____
2._____	4._____	6._____

Disorders of the Pulmonary System

"The two categories of pulmonary disorders cause either chronic long-term changes in respiratory function, such as chronic obstructive pulmonary disease (COPD), or acute changes in respiratory function, such as respiratory distress syndrome (RDS) and acute respiratory failure (ARF)."

Match these pulmonary disorders with the descriptions below.

       A. acute respiratory failure
       B. chronic obstructive pulmonary disease (COPD)
       C. respiratory distress syndrome

1. _____ a progressive and irreversible condition identified by obstruction of air flow; chronic bronchitis, asthma and emphysema

2. _____ sudden absence of respirations, with confusion or unresponsiveness caused by obstructed air flow or failure of the pulmonary gas exchange mechanism

3. _____ a respiratory disorder identified by insufficient respiration and abnormally low levels of circulating oxygen in the blood

PRACTICE EXAM

1. Nutrition-related problems associated with cancer and cancer therapy include all of the following **except**:
   A. taste/smell alterations.
   B. nausea and vomiting.
   C. sneezing and teary eyes.
   D. loss of appetite.

2. A goal for nutrition management of HIV/AIDS may include:
   A. preserving lean body mass and gut function.
   B. minimizing symptoms of malabsorption.
   C. improving sense of well-being and quality of life.
   D. all of the above

3. For patients experiencing respiratory distress syndrome and acute respiratory failure, extra nutrients are required because of:
   A. hypermetabolic conditions.
   B. hypometabolic conditions.
   C. hypoglycemic conditions.
   D. hyperglycemic conditions.

NCLEX Questions

1. Protein-energy malnutrition is the most common problem for patients with cancer. Effects of the malnutrition includes: (PN)
   A. impaired tissue function and repair.
   B. reduced immunocompetence.
   C. better tolerance of treatment.
   D. A and B
   E. A, B, and C

2. Assessment of the nutritional status of a patient with chronic obstructive pulmonary disease is necessary because: (SE)
   A. excessive amounts of energy are used for breathing.
   B. increased risk of malnutrition.
   C. weight loss associated with the disorder includes loss of respiratory muscles and diaphragm.
   D. A and B
   E. A, B, and C

3.   The National Cancer Institute and the American Cancer Society issued   (HP)
     guidelines for cancer prevention. They include all of the following **except**:
     A. eat less high-fiber foods.
     B. eat a variety of foods.
     C. eat fruits and vegetables every day.
     D. reduce fat intake to ≤ 30% of total kcalories.

4.   Fad diets and self-prescribed supplements for patients with HIV/AIDS: (PsN)
     A. may provide an imbalance of nutrients that enhances the immune system.
     B. can be acceptable regardless of risk because the patient believes the diet or
         supplement works.
     C. provide sufficient nutrients.
     D. none of the above

ANSWERS

Important Terms

1. cancer
2. benign neoplasm
3. malignant neoplasm
4. antineoplastic therapy
5. cancer cachexia
6. fractionation
7. neutropenia
8. retrovirus

Applying Content Knowledge

Two concerns to discuss with Meryl include the recommendations of the naturopathic doctor to restrict foods and Meryl's self-imposed caloric restriction of food intake. If the naturopathic plan still provides all of the essential nutrients without the use of supplements and seems to be associated with relief from chemotherapy reactions, the recommendations may be acceptable. To be sure, a registered dietitian and her primary care provider should be notified and should also review the dietary plan to assure adequacy of nutrition. Regarding the patient's caloric restrictions, she should be advised that her body needs sufficient kcalories to heal and maintain her health. Even if her weight increases slightly, it is less stressful on the body than restrictions of kcalories that are usually accompanied by insufficient nutrient intake.

Quick Review

1. Diet is one of the lifestyle and environmental factors that may initiate or reduce risk of cancer in the United States. Certain dietary components such as consumption of fruits and vegetables and higher fiber intakes are associated with a lower risk of developing cancer while consumption of high levels of dietary fat and intake of salt-cured, smoked, and nitrite-preserved foods seem to increase risk of certain cancers. About one third of the cancers in the U.S. may be related to dietary factors.

2. Four possible nutritional interventions for patients with cancer are: for pain, use analgesics 30 to 60 minutes before meals; for nausea, use antiemetic drugs 30 to 60 minutes before meals; give patients and significant other written nutrition guidelines; and encourage patients to eat food, although nutritional supplements may be necessary.

3. Four warning signs are rapid weight loss, gastrointestinal problems, food aversions, and fad diets and/or self-prescribed supplement use.

4. Medical nutrition therapy recommendations are similar for all pulmonary disease disorders. The focus is on consumption of adequate energy and protein to maintain the immune system. The ventilatory drive depends on sufficient protein. The mix of energy nutrients consumed can also affect the carbon dioxide balance and maintain respiratory function. Nonprotein kcalories should be evenly divided between fat and carbohydrate but still not overfeed the patient. If needed enteral and parenteral nutrition may be required to reduce malnutrition.

AIDS and Malnutrition

Physical Symptoms	*Psychosocial Determinants*	*Economic Considerations*
1. anorexia	3. depression	5. loss of job because of illness
2. diarrhea	4. food beliefs	6. excessive health care costs

Nutritional Effects of Cancer Therapy

1. chemotherapy
2. learned food aversions
3. radiation therapy
4. surgery
5. dumping syndrome
6. bone marrow transplantation
7. bacterial and fungal infections

Disorders of the Pulmonary System
1. B   2. A   3. C

Practice Exam
1. C   2. D   3. A

NCLEX Questions
1. D   2. E   3. A   4. D